STUDIES IN POPULATION GENETICS

Edited by **M. Carmen Fusté**

Studies in Population Genetics
Edited by M. Carmen Fusté

Published by InTech
Janeza Trdine 9, 51000 Rijeka, Croatia

Publishing Process Manager Silvia Vlase

Technical Editor Teodora Smiljanic

Cover Designer InTech Design Team

Additional hard copies can be obtained from orders@intechopen.com

Studies in Population Genetics, Edited by M. Carmen Fusté
p. cm.
ISBN 978-953-51-0588-6

For EU product safety concerns:
IN TECH d.o.o., Prolaz Marije Krucifikse Kozulić 3, 51000 Rijeka, Croatia,
info@intechopen.com or visit our website at intechopen.com.

Meet the editor

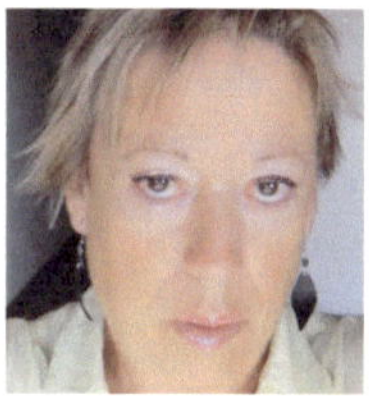

Dr M. Carmen Fusté graduated in Biology at the University of Barcelona, where she completed her PhD in 1980. Since then she has worked in different aspects of Microbiology including bacterial genetics, physiology and bacterial polysaccharide production. Her research in bacterial population genetics began in 1991 with the application of MLEE analysis to the study of different pathogenic and environmental bacteria such as Escherichia coli, Neisseria meningitidis, Haemophilus influenzae, Vibrio cholerae, Pseudomonas stutzeri and Aeromonas. More recently, she has taken advantage of new sequencing techniques to determine the population genetics structure of a group of Aeromonas strains belonging to the "A.hydrophila complex". This work, which has helped clarify this group of species, constitutes one of the chapters of this book.

Contents

Preface

Population geneticists study the genetic composition and variability of natural populations as well as the theories that explain this variability in terms of natural selection, mutation, recombination, genetic drift and gene flow. Population genetics was first developed among eukaryotes in an attempt to reconcile Darwin's theory of evolution by natural selection and Mendelian genetics. When Darwin postulated that natural selection is the main force of evolutionary change, a great controversy was created. As Darwin did not fully understand the inheritance mechanism, he was unable to answer one of the main criticisms of his thesis. If selection is gradually to modify a population, the individuals that constitute this population have to vary, because if all the members are identical, no selection can occur. This controversy would eventually be solved thanks to Mendel's inheritance theory, even though the early Mendelians did not accept an important role for natural selection in evolution.

The foundations of population genetics were established in the 1920s and 1930s when R.A. Fisher, J.B.S. Haldane and S. Wright elaborated mathematical models to explain how Darwin's theory of natural selection (and other evolutionary forces) could modify the genetic composition of a population over time. Since then, research in this field has been mainly focused on eukaryote species and only to a small extent on the prokaryotes, to which population genetics was first applied in the 1970s. The classical analysis of multilocus enzyme electrophoresis (MLEE) has been substituted by new gene sequencing technology, which, being highly reproducible and exportable, has allowed the comparison of data among different laboratories.

The aim of this book has been to reflect the diversity of applications of population genetics. The chapters take a variety of approaches, including general and theoretical, while others report studies on animals, plants and bacteria. Here follows a summary of the different contributions,

Minisatellite markers are revisited, a classic in genetic studies that are back in fashion since their polymorphic nature and high mutation rate allow not only the determination of population divergence over long periods, but also the relatively recent ethnic history of populations. In the search for a comprehensive view of population dynamics, a highly advanced numerical simulation program, which is readily accessible to both students and teachers, is presented. The advantages of using genomic data for population genetics analysis, which has greatly improved our knowledge of mechanisms of mutation and recombination, and adaptation to local environments, is the theme of another contribution. A population genetics study of a Mediterranean species of bat found on the Maltese Islands aims to understand its possible origin and promote its conservation. The goal of another study is to determine the impact of climate change on the evolution and speciation of Brazilian Atlantic Forest Mosquitoes As new techniques for revealing polymorphism have been developed, one chapter comprehensively describes this phenomenon and its use in studying a variety of biological problems, giving extensive examples. An overview of concepts, techniques and empirical data development in plant mating systems is presented in another chapter with a special focus on the evolution of self fertilization in hermaphroditic plants

Finally, a population genetics study sheds light on the doubts about the existence of true species in bacteria. The analysis of several strains included in the "Aeromonas hydrophila species complex" has confirmed that the entities phenotypically described as bacterial species form cohesive groups in which genetic recombination plays a limited role in reducing genetic variation and can therefore be defined as biological species.

Dr M. Carmen Fusté
Department of Health Microbiology and Parasitology, Faculty of Pharmacy,
University of Barcelona, Barcelona,
Spain

1

Piecing the *punicus* Puzzle

Byron Baron
AnGen Labs, Marsascala, Malta

1. Introduction

The occurrence of *Myotis* species in the Mediterranean region has been documented for a very long time. At present, 15 *Myotis* species are known to inhabit the Mediterranean region (Temple & Cuttelod, 2009). However the classification of some of these species has been continuously shifting and somewhat difficult to determine. One such species has been what is now referred to as *Myotis punicus* Felten, 1977 (Castella *et al.*, 2000). Until the late 1990s *Myotis punicus* was generally thought to be an insular variant of either *Myotis myotis* or *Myotis blythii*, mostly because both these species are distributed throughout the Mediterranean region. It was considered to be either a smaller variant of *Myotis myotis* (Gulia, 1913; Ellerman & Morrison-Scott, 1966; Benda & Horácek, 1995), or a larger variant of *Myotis blythii* (Lanza, 1959; Strelkov, 1972; Felten *et al.*, 1977; Bogan *et al.*, 1978; Corbet, 1978). In Malta, some authors also attributed particular individuals to other species including *Myotis daubentoni* (Gulia, 1913), *Myotis capaccinii* (Gulia, 1913) and *Myotis oxygnathus* (Lanfranco, 1969). However, several authors have commented on the differences observed from individuals of *Myotis myotis* and *Myotis blythii* across the rest of their distribution range and expressed doubt as to the correct classification (Strinati, 1951; Strelkov, 1972; Felten *et al.*, 1977; Gaisler, 1983; Menu & Popelard, 1987; Borg *et al.*, 1990; Courtois *et al.*, 1992).

The distinguishing features of *Myotis punicus* were first reported through comparative analyses of morphometric data (Benda & Horácek, 1995; Arlettaz *et al.*, 1997). Cranial morphometrics in conjunction with measurements of forearm and ear length presented a distinct cluster of individuals from the Mediterranean region intermediate in size between *Myotis myotis* and *Myotis blythii*. It was also noted that this intermediate cluster lacked the white spot of hair on the forehead, which is typical of *Myotis blythii* (Arlettaz *et al.*, 1997). Among the distinctive features of *Myotis punicus* are its large size (comparable to *Myotis myotis*), the plagiopatagium (wing membrane) starting at the base of the toes, a lancet shaped tragus and distinct dorsal (light brown) and ventral (white) fur coloration (Dietz & von Helversen, 2004).

2. The appropriate sampling method

However, genetic analysis was required to solve this riddle and obtaining the samples required for such analyses was the first hurdle. In order to carry out research on a protected species such as *Myotis punicus*, which is protected, together with all other European bats under the EUROBATS Agreement (The Agreement on the Conservation of Populations of European Bats, 1994), as well as under local legislation, a sampling permit is required. Permits issued for such research limit the type of sampling that can be carried out and the amount of tissue that can be taken from each individual bat. Most of the genetic analyses carried out on *Myotis* species around the Mediterranean would not have been possible had it not been for the development of a particular non-lethal sampling technique based on skin biopsies (Worthington Wilmer & Barratt, 1996). Before the advent of this technique, the most common methods of obtaining tissue samples from bats for genetic studies had been blood samples, toe clipping (the removal of the smallest digit) or muscle biopsies (Wilkinson and Chapman, 1991) but there were a number of ethical and technical issues associated with such sampling.

The use of this biopsy punch technique for sampling wing and tail membrane was shown to yield sufficient, good quality high molecular weight DNA to carry out most Polymerase Chain Reaction (PCR) based genetic analyses. The main advantages of this sampling technique are that it is quicker and simpler than the previously mentioned sampling methods, can be easily carried out in the field and is applicable to all chiropteran species regardless of size (Worthington Wilmer & Barratt, 1996). Using this method, tissue biopsies are taken from the wing membrane (plagiopatagium) or the tail membrane (uropatagium) using a sterile punch (Stiefel Laboratories) of a diameter that ranges from 2mm to 8mm, the size used being determined by the size and wing area of the bat species being studied. A 3mm punch was reported to yield approximately 15μg of genomic DNA (Worthington Wilmer & Barratt, 1996). This sampling method was originally tested on the species *Pipistrellus pipistrellus* (Barrett *et al.*, 1995) and *Macroderma gigas* (Worthington Wilmer *et al.*, 1994) because they cover most of the size range of michrochiropterans, weighing 5g and 150g respectively. In addition, megachiropteran species were also sampled using this technique (Worthington Wilmer & Barratt, 1996).

This technique was deemed to be safe through follow-up of the sampled bats. The holes in the wing or tail membranes resulting from such biopsies were observed to heal within four weeks in most species (Worthington Wilmer & Barratt, 1996). The presence of tears in bat wings which do not impair the flight capacity of the individual have been frequently observed in the wild, sometimes even as a result of copulation. However in order to be completely safe for the bat, particular attention must be made to select a region of the wing or tail membrane that contains few or no visible blood vessels so that bleeding does not occur and infection is avoided, resulting in faster healing.

3. Piecing the puzzle

With this sampling technique available and proven to be the safest and most effective method available for obtaining genomic DNA from bats, the search into the genetic structure of the Mediteranean *Myotis* species could progress a lot faster. In fact, *Myotis punicus* was proposed as warranting its separate classification at the beginning of the decade on account of studies based on the genetic analyses of cytochrome b (a mitochondrial respiratory gene) and microsatellites (Castella *et al.*, 2000). In this study the authors set out to test the effect of the Strait of Gibraltar as a geographical barrier to gene flow in colonies of *Myotis myotis* between Spain and Morocco. A section of the cytochrome b gene and six microsatellite loci were used in conjunction because, being of mitochondrial and nuclear origin respectively, they provided information regarding the proportion of males and female migrants contributing to the gene pool of a population and shed light onto the phylogenetics of the populations across the Strait of Gibraltar.

The cytochrome b gene is part of the mitochondrial DNA (mtDNA), which means that it is inherited maternally (Avise, 1994) and as such can provide information about the inter-population movements pertinent solely to the females. On the other hand, microsatellites are nuclear markers, which means that they are inherited biparentally (Tautz & Renz, 1984) and thus can be used to follow the movements of both males and females. When comparing microsatellites between two populations, the exchange of mating individuals of just one sex, be it males or females, would be sufficient to homogenise both populations, even if no individuals of the other sex ever leave their native population.

The mtDNA variation observed across the Strait of Gibraltar showed a very weak differentiation between populations on the same side of the Strait because all the mtDNA haplotypes recorded within the Spainish or Moroccan populations were identical or very similar to each other. Concomitantly, almost all the sequence variation present (i.e. 54-59 observed base substitutions over the 600 base pairs of the cytochrome b gene sequenced) was observed when comparing populations across the Strait presenting two groups which are endemic to either side of the Strait of Gibraltar. This dichotomy suggested that this region was inhabited by two genetically distinct groups that have been reproductively isolated for millions of years (Castella *et al.*, 2000). An interesting find was that some cytochrome b haplotypes were only found in one colony, suggesting that females may be more philopatric than males to their natal colonies. In fact, a similar bias of sex dispersal was also proposed as a result of mitochondrial Hypervariable Region I (a control region located within the D-loop of mitochondria) studies carried out on a population of *Myotis myotis* in Germany (Petri *et al.*, 1997). This means that both *Myotis myotis* and *Myotis punicus* are known to exhibit this behaviour.

The findings of the microsatellite analysis supported those from the mtDNA with microsatellite variability being high and evenly distributed among populations from the side of the Strait indicating that colonies from the same side of the Strait were only weakly differentiated from each other. This suggested that there was high nuclear gene flow taking place between the colonies within either region over considerable geographical distances, with a range covering at least 770km, which lead to very weak genetic differentiation between such populations. In contrast, a strong genetic differentiation was apparent across the Strait of Gibraltar. Three of the six microsatellites analysed presented almost no overlap between alleles across the Strait, while the other three microsatellite loci analysed had a more overlapping allelic distribution across the Strait (Castella *et al.*, 2000). The significance of this result to future diagnostic tests was that *Myotis myotis* and *Myotis punicus* could be distinguished using their three unique alleles as well as comparing the allele frequencies for the other three shared loci. Furthermore, the analysis of the same six microsatellite loci in *Myotis blythii* from various locations in Europe and Asia showed that *Myotis blythii* appears to be more closely related to the Spanish populations of *Myotis myotis* than to the Moroccan populations of *Myotis punicus* making it easier to eliminate the possible mix-up caused when using only morphometric comparisons.

Allozyme analysis had been originally used to uncover distinct allelic frequencies for *Myotis* populations from the Mediterranean region (Arlettaz *et al.*, 1997) giving a clear indication that the differences observed from mainland European populations of *Myotis myotis* and *Myotis blythii* where not simply phenotypic variations. Allozymes are allelic variants of enzymes encoded by structural genes. A total of 35 allozyme loci were essayed in these analyses but only 11 of these showed any variability within the three *Myotis* species, having in general either two or three alleles. Some allozymes can be diagnostic as in the case of the ADA and GOT-1 loci, which are fixed for alternative alleles for *Myotis myotis* and *Myotis blythii* in Europe and Asia (Arlettaz, 1995; Arlettaz *et al.*, 1997b). The phylogenetic analysis of these three *Myotis* species in the Mediterranean region using allozymes suggested a closer phylogenetic relationship of *Myotis myotis* with *Myotis punicus* than with *Myotis blythii* although the association was not very strong. These contrast substantially with the phylogenetic results obtained from the combined use of cytochrome b and the six microsatellite loci in which *Myotis myotis* is more closely related to *Myotis blythii* than *Myotis punicus* by a very strong association (Castella *et al.*, 2000).

Additionally, the gathered data was used to understand the process by which *Myotis punicus* established itself and spread in the Mediterranean region. For cytochrome b the authors applied a divergence rate in mammals of 2% per million years (Johns & Avise, 1998) and based on the difference observed between *Myotis myotis* and *Myotis punicus*, which was about 11%, determined that the divergence between these two species must date back to the Pliocene epoch. This means that these species have diverged from a common ancestor around that time and have remained isolated ever since, colonising and spreading along the two sides of the Mediterranean up to their meeting at the Strait of Gibraltar. This hypothesis is supported by the fossil record, given that fossils of typical *Myotis myotis* are known at least since the Pleistocene in Spain (Sevilla, 1989) and the Maltese Islands have been inhabited by *Myotis* species at least since the late Quaternary (Felten *et al.*, 1977), as shown by the fossil records from Ghar Dalam (Storch, 1974). This coincides with the existence of the last land bridge between Europe and North Africa, which was during the last Messinian crisis of 5.5 million years ago, when the greater part of the present-day Mediterranean Sea dried up. Thus dispersal across the Strait of Gibraltar must have been severely limited since the Pliocene. This hypothesis was strengthened when another study of African *Myotis* species showed that the divergence between *Myotis punicus* from *Myotis myotis* and *Myotis blythii* can be traced back to the Pliocene (Stadelmann *et al.*, 2004).

Taking into consideration the long distances *Myotis* species are capable of covering over relatively short periods of time, such as has been shown in *Myotis myotis* females, which are known to cover up to 25km daily between their nursery roosts and feeding grounds (Arlettaz, 1996; Arlettaz, 1999) and annual distances of several hundreds of kilometres between summer and winter roosts (Horácek, 1985; Paz *et al.*, 1986), these species have had ample time to exchange mating individuals between Europe and North Africa especially considering that they have been able to successfully colonise all the major islands of the Mediterranean Sea which could act as stepping stones between the two continents. They have even managed to colonise Mallorca, which is about 200km away from Spain and yet the haplotypes on this island are identical or very similar to those of Spanish populations (Castella *et al.*, 2000).

Both the temporal factor of over 5.5 million years since establishment and the physical ability of *Myotis* species to cover vast distances over both land and sea argue against the hypothesis that 14km of open sea separating Europe from North Africa could have been sufficient as a lone factor to prevent gene flow. Two questions that still remain unanswered however are whether *Myotis myotis* and *Myotis punicus* ever exchange migrants across the Strait of Gibraltar and which routes have been used by these bats to colonise Europe and North Africa. Another more plausible explanation proposed was that of competitive exclusion between *Myotis myotis* and *Myotis punicus* since the niche occupied by *Myotis punicus* in North Africa is very similar to that occupied by *Myotis myotis* in Europe in that both have a diet based on ground-dwelling arthropods such as carabid beetles, ground crickets, scorpions, etc.) (Arlettaz *et al.*, 1997a; Arlettaz, 1999). This does not however explain why *Myotis punicus* is not sympatric with *Myotis blythii* since the latter exploits a completely different niche throughout its distribution range, with a diet that is based principally on grass-dwelling prey such as bush crickets (Arlettaz *et al.*, 1997a; Arlettaz, 1999). Thus, for the moment, the justification for the current distribution of these three sibling species remains open to debate with the historical processes of colonisation and competitive exclusion being the strongest contendants. The only certainty is that to maintain such high levels of genetic differentiation between the populations of the sibling species *Myotis myotis* and *Myotis punicus*, a strong, persistent and ancient barrier preventing gene flow has to be present (Castella *et al.*, 2000).

Over the past ten years the above knowledge about the genetics of *Myotis punicus* has been used to further expand on these analyses and confirm its segregation from *Myotis myotis* and *Myotis blythii* as well as confirm the range of its distribution, which covers the greater part of the Maghreb region from Morocco, through Algeria and Tunisia, up to Tripolitania in north-west Libya and northwards to the European islands of Malta, Corsica and Sardinia (Castella *et al.*, 2000; Mucedda & Nuvoli, 2000; Topál & Ruedi, 2001; Beuneux, 2004; Baron and Vella, 2010; Biollaz *et al.*, 2010).

On the Maltese Islands, *Myotis punicus* has a unique ecological niche because it is the only *Myotis* species and currently their largest resident bat species (Borg, 1998). The Maltese archipelago consists of seven islands covering an area of 316 square kilometres of which only the largest three islands, Malta (245 km^2), Gozo (67 km^2) and Comino (2.8 km^2), are inhabited. The deep karstic caves and extensive garigue spread throughout the archipelago provided the ideal habitat combination for the colonisation of *Myotis punicus*. However, in depth studies to better understand this species in Malta were fuelled by the realisation that incessant human disturbance as a result of urbanisation was leading to dwindling population numbers (Borg, 1998; Baron, 2007; Baron & Vella, 2010).

An allozyme study of the Maltese *Myotis punicus* population was undertaken to compliment data available for *Myotis myotis* and *Myotis blythii* (Ruedi *et al.*, 1990; Arlettaz *et al.* 1997). Using the novel combination of cellulose acetate allozyme electrophoresis with a non-lethal sampling technique (wing biopsy punches), enzyme biochemistry was used to shed light on the allele frequencies at six loci. This study showed that Nei's (1978) Genetic Distance (D) ranged from 0 to 0.047 indicating that the population on the Maltese Islands is a single panmictic unit with an tendency towards becoming isolated mating systems (overall F_{ST} = 0.272) across the territory due to inbreeding as a result of diminishing population numbers. Another interesting outcome of this study was the identification of gene duplication in Glucose Phosphate Isomerase (GPI - 5.3.1.9), which was never reported in *Myotis myotis* and *Myotis blythii* making it a unique species identifier for *Myotis punicus* within this three species complex (Baron & Vella, 2010).

Subsequently the morphometric data collected during the sampling sessions across the Maltese Islands for the allozyme study were amalgamated with those of the previous 20 years to explore the premise of niche expansion in *Myotis punicus* following the extinction of *Rhinolophus ferrumequinum* and shed light onto whether the increase in human disturbance has restricted or promoted variation within the Maltese population. Although the statistics carried out on external characters such as ear length and forearm length showed significant broadening in the value ranges of body size, it was proposed that other more immutable features such as cranial and dentition measurements should be included into such statistical considerations (Baron & Borg, 2011).

Concurrently other researchers were looking in detail at the cranial morphometrics of *Myotis punicus* samples from across the distribution range in greater detail (Evin *et al.*, 2008) and these strengthened the mitochondrial data for *Myotis punicus* (Castella *et al.*, 2000). Using 19 lateral and 29 ventral curvatures and tips present on the skull of *Myotis punicus*, which were mapped as three dimensional co-ordinates, it was possible to obtain a means of identifying *Myotis punicus* from *Myotis myotis* and *Myotis blythii* solely by cranial measurements. The results of this study revealed that the skull shape of *Myotis punicus* completely differs from that of any other *Myotis* in Europe and North Africa (Evin *et al.*, 2008). Apart from that, it was observed that there were morphological differences in the skull shape and size of *Myotis punicus* populations inhabiting the Mediterranean Islands compared to those inhabiting North Africa. This was interpreted as being in accordance with the genetic data available (Castella *et al.*, 2000) which had already indicated the presence of two distinct evolutionary lineages within *Myotis punicus*. The suggested reason for these morphological differences was a strong enough restriction of gene flow between the *Myotis punicus* populations of North Africa and those on the Mediterranean Islands to bring about morphological segregation (also known as demographic independence) (Evin *et al.*, 2008).

However, genetic isolation on its own is not a valid reason for the observed cranial differences. Each phenotypic change is generally driven by a selective pressure presented by the different environments inhabited by the two populations. In bats, diet is known to be an important selective factor acting upon the evolution of cranial morphology (Freeman, 1979; Reduker, 1983; Van Cakenberghe, Herrel & Aguirre, 2002; Aguirre et al., 2003; Dumont & Herrel, 2003). The differences in cranium, teeth and the associated muscles presented by different species are only in part due to the different prey types forming part of a species' diet (Reduker, 1983). Thus when two species have a similar diet it is expected that the cranial morphologies would be similar. This was shown to be the case in *Myotis myotis* which presents greater morphological similarities to *Myotis punicus* than to *Myotis blythii*, which could be the result of morphological convergence due to their similarity in feeding habits (Evin *et al.*, 2008), even though the genetic data had shown *Myotis myotis* to be more closely related to *Myotis blythii*.

Once it was determined that the insular populations of *Myotis punicus* were distinct from those of North Africa, the question arose as to how different the populations on the separate islands were from each other. The cytochrome b gene was sequenced for individuals from roosts across the Maltese Islands in an attempt to isolate SNPs unique to the Maltese population of *Myotis punicus*. Through PCR of the Second Hypervariable Domain (HVII) of the mitochondrial D-loop followed by sequencing, it was determined that only a single haplotype is present on the Maltese Islands (Baron, unpublished). It was recently possible to compare this data with haplotypes isolated from all over the Mediterranean Basin (Biollaz *et al.*, 2010). Interestingly the closest haplotype was found in Tunisia showing that Malta could have been used as a route to the other Mediterranean islands.

In conjunction with the HVII amplification and sequencing, 13 microsatellite loci previously described for *Myotis myotis* (Castella & Ruedi, 2000) were analysed for the Maltese population of *Myotis punicus*. It was thus possible to obtain a reliable data set for a representative number of individuals from across Malta. However, until recently, only limited microsatellite data for *Myotis punicus* was available (Castella *et al.*, 2000). With the availability of microsatellite data from the other Mediterranean Islands to compare with (Biollaz *et al.*, 2010), the microsatellite data collected in Malta could be put to more rigorous evaluation. A permit application has recently been approved to expand this study to sample individuals from as many roosts as possible and obtain a clearer and more complete picture of the variability throughout the Maltese archipelago in an attempt to answer questions related to allele frequency distribution and possible inferences of roost movements.

The mitochondrial and microsatellite haplotypes from the Maltese Islands would not have any meaning had it not been for the detailed work carried out across the Mediterranean region by Biollaz *et al.* (2010). In this study the authors set out to determine the population genetic structure of *Myotis punicus* and current patterns of gene flow between the islands of Corsica and Sardinia and their relationships with North African populations. A combination of mitochondrial and nuclear markers was used to compare levels of gene flow within and between Corsica, Sardinia and North Africa by estimating the contributions of both sexes to the migrant gene pool. Due to the different evolution rates of the selected markers (Chesser & Baker, 1996), it was possible to investigate both recent demographic processes and more remote events in the population history of *Myotis punicus* (Bertorelle & Barbujani, 1995). Based on the proximity between the islands of Corsica and Sardinia and their distance from North Africa, it was expected that a higher genetic differentiation would be present between the populations of North Africa and the two islands than between the insular populations of Corsica and Sardinia.

The theoretical basis of this study is that colonisation of adjacent islands by bats depends in part on the ecological attributes such as dispersal and colonisation abilities of the species and due to this, bat populations on such islands would probably have similar phylogeographical histories as a result of identical colonisation strategies and most probably similar insular geomorphological factors (Trujillo *et al.*, 2002; Pestano *et al.*, 2003; Juste *et al.*, 2004; Salgueiro *et al.*, 2007). However, since the geological history of a region influences the ecology and pattern of diversification of the species, it is the combination of ecological and historical factors of a particular species on a specific island that generates the intraspecific genetic diversity observed between populations on neighbouring islands (Heaney *et al.*, 2005; Roberts, 2006; Heaney, 2007).

The islands of Corsica and Sardinia offer a very interesting view into the dispersal of *Myotis punicus* because they have common geological (Meulenkamp & Sissingh, 2003) and faunal assemblage histories (Vigne, 1992; Ferrandini & Salotti, 1995; van der Made, 1999; Marra, 2005; Sondaar & Van der Geer, 2005). In addition to this, after the Messinian salinity crisis, which occurred 5.5 million years ago (Krijgsman *et al.*, 1999), Corsica and Sardinia were isolated from the mainland by Pliocene flooding (van der Made et al., 2006), which gave rise to endemic species (Carranza & Amat, 2005) but then during the Pleistocene glaciations, the lowering in sea level provided periods of intermittent contact during which faunal exchanges could have possibly occurred (Lanza, 1972; Lanza, 1983; Caloi *et al.*, 1986; van Andel & Tzedakis, 1996).

The mitochondrial analysis of part of the HVII of the mitochondrial D-loop was carried out using primers previously tested on *Myotis myotis* (Fumagalli *et al.*, 1996; Castella *et al.*, 2001). Sequencing of the HVII region revealed 26 different haplotypes (3 haplotypes in Corsica, 13 in Sardinia, 3 in Morocco and 7 in Tunisia). The sequenced region contained a total of 38 variables sites, of which 31 were present more than once. The haplotypes segregated into three main groups - corresponding to the combined samples from the islands of Corsica and Sardinia, the samples from the region around Tunisia and the samples from across Morocco. About 15 mutations separated Corsica and Sardinia from Tunisia and Morocco and the latter two between themselves. Interestingly, no haplotypes were shared between the islands since the insular populations were separated by at least one mutation. The results also suggested that the Corsican haplotypes are derived from the most represented Sardinian haplotype, which was found in almost half the sampled Sardinian individuals. This means that the population inhabiting Corsica most probably crossed over from Sardinia. Similarly in Morocco, the great majority of samples were represented by a single haplotype. Thus overall, haplotype diversity and nucleotide diversity were lower in the populations of Morocco and Corsica than in those of Tunisia and Sardinia (Biollaz *et al.*, 2010). The mitochondrial data was also used to estimate the time of divergence of the insular populations. These analyses indicated that the Sardinian population separated from the common ancestor population in North Africa during the early Pleistocene while the Corsican populations diverged much later, during the mid-Pleistocene. These results support the hypothesis that the colonisation of the Mediterranean islands by *Myotis punicus* occurred in a stepping-stone manner.

The microsatellite analyses involving the use of seven loci were amplified and analysed using primers originally designed for *Myotis myotis* (Castella & Ruedi, 2000). The microsatellite results confirmed the segregation obtained through the mitochondrial analysis, with no differentiation being observed for all seven microsatellite loci between the insular populations or between the populations of North Africa. On the other hand, there were no shared haplotypes between the populations of North Africa, Sardinia and Corsica (Biollaz et al., 2010).

The data from these two sets of molecular markers was used to understand the exchange of individual between the islands of Corsica and Sardinia. The authors focused solely on the exchange of individuals between the islands because of the geographical distances involved. While Sardinia is separated from North Africa by 200km of open water, the islands of Corsica and Sardinia are separated by the Strait of Bonifacio, which is just 11km. Mitochondrial and nuclear analyses both suggested that male and female *Myotis punicus* moved freely within Corsica and Sardinia and thus appeared to be strong dispersers compared with the populations in North Africa. The authors suggest that the discrepancy between the populations of North Africa and those on Corsica and Sardinia could be due to a non-equilibrium situation on the islands with contemporary gene flow being masked by the fact that these populations are expanding or recently established from a common source population (Whitlock, 1992). On the other hand, despite the apparent high dispersal ability, dispersal between Corsica and Sardinia is virtually non-existent. Open water seems to represent an almost unsurpassable barrier that drastically hampers gene flow between Corsica, Sardinia and North Africa irrespective of the distance. As a result of this, *Myotis punicus* populations inhabiting Corsica and Sardinia appear to be completely isolated (Biollaz *et al.*, 2010).

The hypothesis that Corsica might have been colonised from Sardinia and the strong bottleneck resulting from such a colonisation event could explain the lower mitochondrial diversity observed in the *Myotis punicus* population of Corsica. Small insular populations, due to the limited carrying capacity of such islands, tend to be more susceptible to extinction and drift and as a result show less variability than on larger islands which can support a more extensive genetic variability (Johnson *et al.*, 2000). Corsica is smaller than Sardinia and most distant from the North African source population. Moreover, caves are a rare habitat which can be found exclusively in the north of the island (Courtois *et al.*, 1997), while Sardinia is larger and more karstic, with more potentially suitable caves and foraging habitats. Also, while the population of *Myotis punicus* in Corsica is currently estimated at around 3000 individuals with four nursery colonies (Beuneux, 2004), that in Sardinia consists of 19 large nursery colonies (Mucedda *et al.*, 1999). Therefore, the smaller population size of Corsica contains a lower genetic diversity, especially since there is no immigration from Sardinia. Compared with the pooled population of North Africa, Corsica and Sardinia harbour significantly lower allelic richness as well as observed and expected heterozygosities (Biollaz *et al.*, 2010). The authors suggest that such genetic features could reflect recent population crashes or a bottleneck during the colonisation of these islands, reducing the effective population size (Frankham, 1997; Knopp *et al.*, 2007).

The reasoning behind the colonisation of Corsica from Sardinia is based on the availability of land bridges during subsequent Pleistocene glaciations which brought about the lowering of sea level and the exposure of previously submerged land (Rohling *et al.*, 1998). The geographical distances between Mediterranean islands and the surrounding mainland were thus reduced and with the emergence of land bridges between some islands, it became easier for species to explore and colonise new territories and one of the species that took advantage of this situation was *Myotis punicus*. The population spread out slowly from North Africa and extended all the way up to Corsica in stages. Once the glaciation periods ended and the water levels rose again the colonising populations were isolated and this would explain the strong reduction of gene flow observed in both mitochondrial and genomic markers.

Interestingly, despite the presence of no water barriers in North Africa, a strong mitochondrial differentiation was revealed between the nursery colonies of *Myotis punicus* in Tunisia and Morocco. This contrasts strongly with the phylogeographical pattern observed in European *Myotis myotis*, which present a main haplotype spanning from the south of Spain to Poland and Greece. The pattern of mitochondrial haplotype uniformity across Europe in *Myotis myotis* was explained by a post-glacial recolonisation from a single Spanish glacial refugium (Ruedi & Castella, 2003). The huge divergence between the populations of Tunisia and Morocco suggests that these two populations have in some way been isolated since the Pleistocene. In fact, despite the current nuclear gene flow (which is due to male-biased dispersal), no female exchange seems to have occurred since then. Thus it was proposed that the low haplotype diversity due to isolation could have been enhanced by a combination of the populations in Morocco being confined to the High Atlas Mountains and the philopatric behaviour of *Myotis punicus* females (Biollaz *et al.*, 2010). This is not an isolated case of divergence in North Africa. Similar divergence between eastern and western lineages in North Africa have been previously documented in species such as in white-toothed shrews, *Crocidura russula* (Brändli *et al.*, 2005), in tree frogs, *Hyla* spp. (Stöck *et al.*, 2008), and in spur-thighed tortoises, *Testudo graeca* (Fritz *et al.*, 2009). This demonstrates that a strong barrier, possibly driven by climatic fluctuations during the Pleistocene, has affected the distribution of a number of species lineages in this region (Biollaz *et al.*, 2010).

A by-product of the research into the *Myotis punicus* population of the Maltese Islands was the setting up of a technique for the preparation of *Myotis punicus* cell lines. The testing of three mitochondrial regions and thirteen microsatellites for each bat sampled required more DNA than was being collected per individual as stipulated by the legal permit for protected species issued for the project, especially in the cases where sequencing did not give conclusive results and the sample had to be retested for one or more loci. To supplement the need for more DNA the two options available were either to bulk up the DNA extracted from each biopsy punch using whole genome amplification or else increase the amount of cellular material used for the DNA extraction. The latter was opted for and a cell culture project was set up in which transient cell lines were created for as many individuals as possible. The success rate of this culture effort was 37% due to a number of limiting factors. The prime difficulty was antibiotic resistant fungal infections that had survived the short wash step in 70% ethanol and that had transferred into the culture medium from the wing membrane. The second most common setback was that samples did not present a large enough seeding surface and died before enough cells had grown out, onto the plastic surface, to be able to sustain a cell population. In addition to growing primary cultures of fibroblasts several attempts were made to obtain an immortalised (permanent) *Myotis punicus* cell line. The difficulty in transfecting and immortalising primary cells is well known and although the transfection and selection processes were successful, no immortalised cell line has as yet been achieved. The benefit of having available such cell cultures greatly outweighs the effort put into the set up, optimisation and maintenance required and the use of this technique for the production of transient cultures in vitro can be applied to any line of chiropteran genetic conservation research (Baron, in preparation).

4. Conclusion

Thus, over the past eleven years, the resident *Myotis* species of the Maltese Islands has gone from being considered a small, unimportant population of either *Myotis myotis* or *Myotis blythii*, about which very little was known, to a key population in the understanding of how a species unique to the Mediteranean has spread from North Africa towards the European islands by a stepping-stone mechanism through allozyme, mitochondrial and microsatellite analyses and has served as a driving force in the development of a cell culture technique for chiropteran conservation genetics.

In the end, every research question answered adds another piece to this puzzle but there are dozens of questions still unanswered regarding the *Myotis punicus* population on the Maltese Islands such as: Is there an exchange of individuals with other populations of the Mediterranean region? If yes, where from and where to? how often? and what is the driving force for these migrations? If not, is the aquatic barrier the only factor limiting this exchange? Are there any unique genetic markers to this insular population of *Myotis punicus*? If inbreeding becomes a critical issue, would it be possible to bring in individuals to boost numbers? and which would be the best population to bring them from?

As more advanced laboratory techniques become available, more questions will be answered, adding even more pieces to this puzzle and other questions as yet unasked might eventually find themselves forming part of this ever-growing puzzle for future scientists to solve.

5. References

Aguirre, L.F., Herrel, A., van Damme, R., & Matthysen, E. (2003). The implications of food hardness for diet in bats. *Functional Ecology* 17: 201–212.

Arlettaz, R. (1995). Ecology of the Sibling Mouse-Eared Bats (*Myotis myotis* and *Myotis blythii*): Zoogeography, Niche, Competition, and Foraging. Horus Publishers, Martigny, Switzerland.

Arlettaz, R. (1996). Feeding behaviour and foraging strategy of free-living Mouse-eared bats, *Myotis myotis* and *Myotis blythii*. *Animal Behaviour*, 51: 1-11.

Arlettaz, R. (1999). Habitat selection as a major resource partitioning mechanism between the two sympatric sibling bat species *Myotis myotis* and *Myotis blythii*. *Journal of Animal Ecology*, 68: 460-471.

Arlettaz, R., Perrin, N., & Hausser, J. (1997a). Trophic resource partitioning and competition between the two sibling bat species *Myotis myotis* and *Myotis blythii*. *Journal of Animal Ecology*, 66: 897-911.

Arlettaz, R., Ruedi, M., Ibañez, C., Pameirim, J., & Hausser, J. (1997b). A new perspective on the zoogeography of the sibling mouse-eared bat species *Myotis myotis* and *Myotis blythii* : morphological, genetical and ecological evidence. *J. Zool., Lond.* 242: 45-62.

Avise, J.C. (1994). Molecular markers, natural history and evolution. Chapman & Hall, New York.

Baron, B. (2007). A look at the Chiropteran Fauna of the Maltese Islands: Towards an effective Action Plan for their conservation. *Xjenza* 12 (2007): 1-9.

Baron, B., & Borg, J.J. (2011). Evidence of niche expansion in the *Myotispunicus*(*Mammalia Chiroptera*) of the Maltese Islands. *Naturalista sicil.*, S. IV, 35 (2): 3-13.

Baron, B., & Vella, A. (2010). A preliminary analysis of the population genetics of *Myotis punicus* in the Maltese Islands. *Hystrix It. J. Mamm.* (n.s.) 21(1) (2010): 65-72.

Barrett, E.M., Bruford, M.W., Burland, T.M., Jones, G., Racey, P.A., & Wayne, R.K. (1995). Characterization of mitochondrial DNA variability within the michrochiropteran genus *Pipistrellus*: Approaches and applications. *Symposium of the Zoological Society of London*, 67: 377-386.

Barrett, E.M., Deaville, R., Burland, T.M., Bruford, M.W., Jones, G., Racey, P.A., & Wayne, R.K. (1997). DNA answers the call of pipistrelle bat species. *Nature*, 387: 138-139.

Benda, P., & Horácek, I. (1995). Biometrics of *Myotis myotis* and *Myotis blythi*. *Myotis* 32-33: 45-55.

Bertorelle, G. & Barbujani, G. (1995) Analysis of DNA diversity by spatial autocorrelation. *Genetics*, 140: 811–819.

Beuneux, G. (2004). Morphometrics and ecology of *Myotis* cf. *punicus* (Chiroptera, Vespertilionidae) in Corsica. *Mammalia* 68 (4): 269-273.

Biollaz, F., Bruyndonckx, N., Beuneux, G., Mucedda, M., Goudet, J., & Christe, P. (2010). Genetic isolation of insular populations of the Maghrebian bat, *Myotis punicus*, in the Mediterranean Basin. *Journal of Biogeography*, Volume 37, Issue 8, 1557-1569.

Bogan, M.A., Setzer, H.W., Findley, J.S., & Wilson, D.E. (1978). Phenetics of *Myotis blythii* in Morocco. In: Proceedings of the Fourth International Bat Research Conference, Nairobi, pp. 217-230.

Borg, J., Fiore, M., Violani, C., & Zava, B. (1990). Observations on the Chiropterofauna of Gozo, Maltese Islands. *Boll. Mus. Reg. Nat. Torino* 8: 501-515.

Borg, J.J. (1998). The Lesser Mouse-eared Bat *Myotis blythii punicus* Felten, 1977 in Malta. Notes on status, morphometrics, movements, and diet (Chiroptera, Vespertilionidae). *Naturalista Siciliano* 22 (3-4): 365-374.

Brändli, L., Handley, L.J.L., Vogel, P., & Perrin, N. (2005). Evolutionary history of the greater white-toothed shrew (Crocidura russula) inferred from analysis of mtDNA, Y, and X chromosome markers. *Molecular Phylogenetics and Evolution*, 37: 832–844.

Caloi, L.T., Kotsakis, M., & Palombo, R. (1986). La fauna vertebrati terrestri del Pleistocene delle isole del Mediterraneo. *Geologica Romana*, 25: 235–256.

Carranza, S., & Amat, F. (2005). Taxonomy, biogeography and evolution of Euproctus (Amphibia: Salamandridae), with the resurrection of the genus Calotriton and the description of a new endemic species from the Iberian Peninsula. *Zoological Journal of the Linnean Society*, 145: 555–582.

Castella, V., & Ruedi, M. (2000). Characterization of highly variable microsatellite loci in the bat *Myotis myotis* (Chiroptera: Vespertilionidae). *Molecular Ecology*, 9, 993-1011.

Castella, V., & Ruedi, M. (2000). Characterization of highly variable microsatellite loci in the bat *Myotis myotis* (Chiroptera: Vespertilionidae). *Molecular Ecology*, 9: 1000- 1002.

Castella, V., Ruedi, M., & Excoffier, L. (2001). Contrasted patterns of mitochondrial and nuclear structure among nursery colonies of the bat *Myotis myotis*. *Journal of Evolutionary Biology*, 14: 708–720.

Castella, V., Ruedi, M., Excoffier, L., Ibanez, C., Arlettez, R., & Hausser, J. (2000). Is the Gibraltar Strait a barrier to gene flow for the bat *Myotis myotis* (Chiroptera: Vespertilionidae). *Molecular Ecology*, 9, 1761-1772.

Chesser, R.K. & Baker, R.J. (1996) Effective sizes and dynamics of uniparentally and diparentally inherited genes. *Genetics*, 144: 1225–1235.

Corbet, G.B. (1978). The mammals of the Palaearctic Region: a taxonomic review. Cornell University Press, London.

Courtois, J.Y., Faggio, G., & Salotti, M. (1992). Chiroptères de Corse. Actualisation des cartes de repartition et revision du statut des espèces troglophiles. Biguglia: Corsica Stampa.

Courtois, J.Y., Mucedda, M., Salotti, M., & Casale, A. (1997). Deux îles, deux peuplements: comparaison des populations de Chiropte`res troglophiles de Corse et de Sardaigne. *Arvicola*, 9: 15–18.

Dietz, C., & von Helversen, O. (2004). Illustrated identification key to the bats of Europe. Electronic Publication. Version 1.0. released 15.12.2004. Tuebingen & Erlangen (Germany).

Dumont, E.R., & Herrel, A. (2003). The effects of gape angle and bite point on bite force in bats. *The Journal of Experimental Biology* 206: 2117-2123.

Ellerman, J.R., & Morrison-Scott, T.C.S. (1966). Checklist of Palaearctic and Indian Mammals, 1758-1946. Alden Press, Oxford.

Evin, A., Baylac, M., Ruedi, M., Mucedda, M., & Pons, J.M. (2008). Taxonomy, skull diversity and evolution in a species complex of *Myotis* (Chiroptera: Vespertilionidae): a geometric morphometric appraisal. *Biological Journal of the Linnean Society*, 95: 529-538.

Felten, H., Spitzenberger, F., & Storch, G. (1977). Zur Kleinsäugerfauna West-Anatoliens. Teil IIIa. *Senckenberg. Biol.* 58: 1-44.

Ferrandini, J., & Salotti, M. (1995). Discovery of considerable upper Pleistocene and Holocene fossil fillings in the karst of Oletta region (Corsica). *Geobios*, 28: 117-124.

Frankham, R. (1997). Do island populations have less genetic variation than mainland populations? *Heredity*, 78: 311-327.

Freeman, P. (1979). Specialized insectivory: beetle-eating and moth-eating molossid bats. *Journal of Mammalogy* 60: 467- 479.

Fritz, U., Harris, D.J., Fahd, S., Rouag, R., Martínez, E.G., Casalduero, A.G., Široký, P., Kalboussi, M., Jdeidi, T.B., & Hundsdörfer, A.K. (2009). Mitochondrial phylogeography of Testudo graeca in the Western Mediterranean: old complex divergence in North Africa and recent arrival in Europe. *Amphibia-Reptilia*, 30: 63-80.

Fumagalli, L., Taberlet, P., Favre, L., & Hausser, J. (1996). Origin and evolution of homologous repeated sequences in the mitochondrial DNA control region of shrews. *Molecular Biology and Evolution*, 13: 31-46.

Gaisler, J. (1983). Nouvelles données sur les Chiropteres du nord algérien. Mammalia 47: 359-369.

Gulia, G. (1913). Uno Sguardo alla Zoologia delle Isole Maltesi. IX International Congress of Zoology, Monaco, March 1913, Pages: 545-555.

Heaney, L.R. (2007). Is a new paradigm emerging for oceanic island biogeography? *Journal of Biogeography*, 34: 753-757.

Heaney, L.R., Walsh, J.S., & Peterson, A.T. (2005). The roles of geological history and colonization abilities in genetic differentiation between mammalian populations in the Philippine archipelago. *Journal of Biogeography*, 32: 229-247.

Horácek, I. (1985). Population ecology of *Myotis myotis* in Central Bohemia (Mammalia: Chiroptera). Acta Universitas Carolinae - Biologica, 8: 161-267.

Johns, G.C., & Avise, J.C. (1998). A comparative summary of genetic distances in the vertebrates from the mitochondrial Cytochrome b gene. *Molecular Biology and Evolution*, 15: 1481-1490.

Johnson, K.P., Adler, F.R., & Cherry, J.L. (2000). Genetic and phylogenetic consequences of island biogeography. *Evolution*, 54: 387-396.

Juste, J., Ibáñez, C., Muñoz, J., Trujillo, D., Benda, P., Karatas, A., & Ruedi, M. (2004). Mitochondrial phylogeography of the long-eared bats (*Plecotus*) in the Mediterranean Palaearctic and Atlantic Islands. *Molecular Phylogenetics and Evolution*, 31: 1114–1126.

Knopp, T., Cano, J.M., Crochet, P.A., & Merila, J. (2007). Contrasting levels of variation in neutral and quantitative genetic loci on island populations of moor frogs (*Rana arvalis*). *Conservation Genetics*, 8: 45–56.

Krijgsman, W., Hilgen, F.J., Raffi, I., Sierro, F.J., & Wilson, D.S. (1999). Chronology, causes and progression of the Messinian salinity crisis. *Nature*, 400: 652–655.

Lanfranco, G. (1969). Maltese Mammals (Central Mediterranean). Progress press, Malta, Pp: 1-28.

Lanza, B. (1959). Chiroptera Blumenbach, 1774 (pp. 187-473). In: Toschi A., and Lanza B. Fauna d'Italia, Vol. IV, Mammalia, generalità, Insectivora, Chiroptera; Bologna; Ed. Calderini, pp. 485.

Lanza, B. (1972). The natural history of the Cerbicale Islands (southeastern Corsica) with particular reference to their herpetofauna. *Natura Bresciana*, 63, 185–202.

Lanza, B. (1983). Ipotesi sulle origini del popolamento erpetologico della Sardegna. *Lavori della Societa Italiana di Biogeografia*, 8: 723–744.

Marra, A.C. (2005). Pleistocene mammals of Mediterranean islands. *Quaternary International*, 129: 5–14.

Menu, H. & Popelard, J.B. (1987). Utilisation des caractères dentaires pour la déterermination des vespertilionidés de l'ouest européen. *Rinolophe* 4: 1-88.

Meulenkamp, J.E., & Sissingh, W. (2003). Tertiary palaeogeography and tectonostratigraphic evolution of the Northern and Southern Peri-Tethys platforms and the intermediate domains of the African–Eurasian convergent plate boundary zone. *Palaeogeography, Palaeoclimatology, Palaeoecology*, 196: 209–228.

Mucedda, M., & Nuvoli, T. (2000). Indagine biometrica sul "grande Myotis" (Chiroptera, Vespertilionidae) della Grotta Sa Rocca Ulari (Borutta) e di alter località della Sardegna. *Sardegna Speleol.* 17: 46-51.

Mucedda, M., Bertelli, M.L., & Pidinchedda, E. (1999). Risultati di 6 anni di censimento dei pipistrelli in Sardegna. Atti del primo convegno italiano sui chirotteri (ed. by G. Dondini, O. Papalini and S. Vergari), pp. 105–114. Proceedings of the First Italian Bat Congress, Castell'Azzara (Grosseto).

Nei, M. (1978). Estimation of Average Heterozygosity and genetic Distance from a small number of individuals. *Genetics* 89: 583-590 July, 1978

Paz, de O., Fernandez, R., & Benzal, J. (1986). El anillamiento de Quiropteros en el centro de la peninsula iberica durante el period 1977-86. *Boletin de la Estacion Central de Ecologia*, 30: 113-138.

Pestano, J., Brown, R.P., Suárez, N.M., Benzal, J., & Fajardo, S. (2003). Intraspecific evolution of Canary Island Plecotine bats, based on mtDNA sequences. *Heredity*, 90: 302–307.

Petri, B., Pääbo, S., Von Haeseler, A., & Tautz, D. (1997). Paternity assessment and population subdivision in a natural population of the Larger Mouse eared bat *Myotis myotis*. *Ecology*, 6: 235-242.

Reduker, D.W. (1983). Functional analysis of the masticatory apparatus in two species of *Myotis*. *Journal of Mammogy* 64: 277–286.

Roberts, T.E. (2006). Multiple levels of allopatric divergence in the endemic Philippine fruit bat Haplonycteris fischeri (Pteropodidae). *Biological Journal of the Linnean Society*, 88: 329–349.

Rohling, E.J., Fenton, M., Jorissen, F.J., Bertrand, P., Ganssen, G., & Caulet, J.P. (1998). Magnitudes of sea-level low stands of the past 500,000 years. *Nature*, 394: 162–165.

Ruedi, M., & Castella, V. (2003). Genetic consequences of the ice ages on nurseries of the bat Myotis myotis: a mitochondrial and nuclear survey. *Molecular Ecology*, 12: 1527–1540.

Ruedi, M., Arlettaz, R., & Maddalena, T. (1990). Distinction morphologique et biochimique de deux espèce jumelles de chauves souris: *Myotis myotis* (Bork.) et *Myotis blythii* (Tomes) (Mammalia; Vespertilionidae). *Mammalia* 54: 3, 415-429.

Salgueiro, P., Ruedi, M., Coelho, M.M., & Palmeirim, J.M. (2007). Genetic divergence and phylogeography in the genus *Nyctalus* (Mammalia, Chiroptera): implications for population history of the insular bat *Nyctalus azoreum*. *Genetica*, 130: 169–181.

Sevilla, P. (1989). Quaternary fauna of bats in Spain: Paleoecologic and biogeographic interest. In: *European Bat Research 1987* (eds. Hanak, V., Horácek, I., & Gaisler, J.), pp. 349-355. Charles University Press, Praha, Tchechia.

Sondaar, P.Y., & Van der Geer, A.A.E. (2005). Evolution and extinction of Plio-Pleistocene island ungulates. *Les ongulés holarctiques du Pliocène et du Pléistocene* (ed. by E. Crégut-Bonnoure), pp. 241–256. Maison de la Géologie, Paris.

Stadelmann, B., Jacobs, D.S., Schoeman, C., & Ruedi, M. (2004). Phylogeny of African *Myotis* bats (Chiroptera, Vespertilionidae) inferred from cytochrome b sequences. *Acta Chiropterologica*, 6: 177–192.

Storch G. (1974). Quartare Fledermaus-Faunen von der Insel Malta. *Senckenbergiana lethaea* 55 (1/5): 407-434.

Stöck, M., Dubey, S., Klütsch, C., Litvinchuk, S.N., Scheidt, U., & Perrin, N. (2008). Mitochondrial and nuclear phylogeny of circum-Mediterranean tree frogs from the Hyla arborea group. *Molecular Phylogenetics and Evolution*, 49: 1019– 1024.

Strelkov, P.P. (1972). Myotis blythii (Tomes, 1857): Distribution, geographical variability and differences from *Myotis myotis* (Borkhausen, 1797). *Acta Theriol.* 17: 355-380. (In Russian).

Strinati, P. (1951). Note sure les chauves-souris du Maroc. *Mammalia* 15: 23-31.

Tautz D., & Renz, M. (1984). Simple sequences are ubiquitous repetitive components of eukaryotic genomes. *Nucleic Acid Research*, 12: 4127-4138.

Temple, H.J., & Cuttelod, A. (Compilers). 2009. *The Status and Distribution of Mediterranean Mammals*. Gland, Switzerland and Cambridge, UK: IUCN. vii+32pp. Available at: http://cmsdata.iucn.org/downloads/mediteranean_mammals_web2.pdf (cited on 13th August 2011).

Topál, G., & Ruedi, M. (2001). *Myotis blythii* (Tomes, 1857) - Kleines Mausohr, in Handbuch der Säugetiere Europas. Band 4/I (Fledertiere). Ed. F. Krapp, Aula-Verlag, Wiebelsheim: 209-215.

Trujillo, D., Ibáñez, C., & Juste, J. (2002). A new subspecies of *Barbastella barbastellus* (Mammalia: Chiroptera: Vespertilionidae) from the Canary Islands. *Revue Suisse de Zoologie*, 109: 543–550.

van Andel, T.H., & Tzedakis, P.C. (1996). Palaeolithic landscapes of Europe and environs, 150,000–25,000 years ago. *Quaternary Science Reviews*, 15: 481–500.

Van Cakenberghe, V., Herrel, A., & Aguirre, L.F. (2002). Evolutionary relationships between cranial shape and diet in bats (Mammalia: Chiroptera). In: Aerts P, ed. *Topics in functional and ecological vertebrate morphology*. Maastricht: Shaker Publishing, 205–236.

van der Made, J. (1999). Biogeography and stratigraphy of the Mio-Pleistocene mammals of Sardinia and the description of some fossils. *Deinsea* (Rotterdam), 7: 337–360.

Vigne, J.D. (1992). Zooarchaeology and the biogeographical history of the mammals of Corsica and Sardinia since the last ice age. *Mammal Review*, 22: 87–96.

Whitlock, M.C. (1992) Temporal fluctuations in demographic parameters and the genetic variance among populations. *Evolution*, 46: 608–615.

Wilkinson, G.S., & Chapman, A.M. (1991). Length and sequence variation in evening bat d-loop mtDNA. *Genetics*, 128: 607-617.

Worthington Wilmer, J., & Barratt, E. (1996). A non-lethal method of tissue sampling for genetic studies of chiropterans. *Bat Research News*, 37:1–3.

Worthington Wilmer, J.M., Moritz, C., Hall, L., & Toop, J. (1994). Extreme population structuring in the threatened ghost bat, *Macroderma gigas*: Evidence from mitochondrial DNA. *Proceedings of the Royal Society, London*. Series B, 257: 193-198.

2

The Evolution of Plant Mating System: Is It Time for a Synthesis?

Cheptou Pierre-Olivier
UMR 5175 CEFE
Centre d'Ecologie Fonctionnelle et Evolutive (CNRS), Montpellier Cedex, France

1. Introduction

Diversity is the rule in living organisms. While this diversity is manifest at the various levels of the life tree, the diversity in the vegetable kingdom is probably the most apparent form, as revealed by the high diversity of plant morphologies and life histories even at small spatial scale. Since the first investigations in plant biology, botanists have always focused on the high variation of reproductive systems in plants and the floral diversity (forms and colors) in higher plants is one of the most obvious forms of variation. This has provided the basis for discriminating and classifying plants. In the 18th century, variation in sexual structures of plants has thus provided the basis for the Linnaean classification. Interestingly, such variation reveals variation and adaptation of the mating system and results from evolutionary processes in the phylogeny. Moreover, mating systems are central in population biology first because it ensures the maintenance (and eventually the growth) of populations and second because it shapes the transmission of phenotypic traits via the transmission of the hereditary material, thus conditioning evolutionary processes.

If the diversity of plant reproductive systems and floral morphologies have intrigued naturalists for a long time, botanic studies have long been only descriptive, without any evolutionary interpretation for the rise of such diversity. The first evolutionary interpretation has been proposed by Darwin who devoted three volumes on plants reproductive biology (Darwin, 1867; Darwin, 1876; Darwin, 1877). Pollination processes and the dependence to pollen vectors was the central selective force in Darwin's view. The rise of mendelian laws and more recently population genetics, particularly Sir Ronald Fisher's work in the 1940's, have laid the foundation for a solid theoretical framework, based on gene dynamics. In constrast, the botanical tradition has been developed in a more empirical way. These two historical traditions have given birth to two different approaches that have remained relatively separated until recently (Uyenoyama et al. 1993). In the last ten years, the rapprochement is however perceptible (Barrett, 2008). Interestingly, plant mating system studies is good example of fruitfull interaction between field data, theory and experiments. Field observations of flowering plants, interactions with pollinators have provided an important corpus of data. Also, mating system theory is an active field of research addressing major issues in evolutionary biology such as kin selection, the effect of deleterious mutations or mutual interactions. Finally, plant mating system is an area where the experimental approach to test specific hypotheses has been succesful thanks to suitable tools and techniques. As a matter of example, self-fertilization can be precisely measured under natural conditions thanks to genetic markers, it can also be manipulated in laboratory thus allowing to test adaptive hypotheses.

In this review, I will present an overview of concepts, techniques and empirical data developed in plant mating system. Plant mating system encompasses various subfields such as the evolution of separate sexes, asexuality, the maintenance of sexual polymorphism in populations and the evolution in inbreeding regime. Because the evolution of self-fertilisation has been intensively studied and because hermaphroditism is widespread in plants, my chapter will focus mainly on the evolution of self-fertilisation in hermaphroditic plants.

2. Inbreeders and outbreeders in plants

2.1 The diversity of flowering plants

In higher plants, the flower is the fundamental unit for sexual reproduction. While the perfect flower is hermaphroditic, bearing both male (stamen) and female (pistil) functions, variations around the perfect type are theoretically possible. Some individuals may bear only female flower while other individuals bear male flower. Also, different type of flowers can coexist within individuals. These variations may be predicted by various combinations and it is important to note that most of them have been found in nature (Richard 1986). For example, dioecy corresponds to two types of individuals within populations: male bearing male flowers and female bearing female flowers. On this basis, up to seven types of sexual systems have been found in natural populations (see table 1). Among them, hermaphroditism where a single sexual type occurs in populations is by far the most widespread sexual types in higher plants representing more than 70% (Yampolsky and Yampolsky, 1922). It is worth noting that hermaphroditism also exists in many animal phyla (Jarne 1993) though it has mostly been studied in plants.

One sexual type	%	*Two sexual types*	%
Hermaphroditism (⚥)	72	Dioecy (♂ + ♀)	4
Monoecy (♂-♀)	5	Gynodioecy (♀ + ⚥)	7
Andromonoecy (♂-⚥)	1.7	Androdioecy (♂ + ⚥)	rare
Gynomonoecy (♀-⚥)	2.8		

Table 1. Classification of plant sexual types based (1) on the number of sexual types in the population and (2) on the number of sexes per sexual type. Hyphens in the first column symbolizes flower types in the same individual and the sign "plus" represents the occurrence of several sexual types in populations.

The evolution of separate sexes has often been considered as a way to avoid inbreeding (Bawa, 1980) but Charnov (1976) has provided another important argument based on resource allocation. Even in absence of self-fertilisation in hermaphrodites, Charnov (1976) showed that dioecy may be selectively advantageous depending on ressource trade-offs between male and female functions. The question of the maintenance of females in gynodioecious plants or symmetrically males in androdioecious plants has been subject to important debate. Both theoretical models and empirical studies have shown that gynodiecy is evolutionary stable (e.g. *Thymus vulgaris*; Gouyon and Couvet, 1988). Interestingly, empirical data have revealed that the determinism of sexual types implies cytaplasmic genes coding for male sterility (favouring female transmission) and nuclear genes restoring male fertility. Theoretical studies have confirmed that nucleo-cytoplasmic allowed gynodioecy to evolve on a large range of parameters and models have revealed a male/female conflict. While androdioecy may seem similar, theoretical studies have shown that the conditions for its stability are narrow, which lead some authors to doubt about the existence of "true androdioecy" in plants (Charlesworth, 1984). A recent study by Saumitou-laprade et al. (2009) on *Phyllirea angustifolia* (Oleaceae) has demonstrated first that the species was functionally androdioecious and second, that self-incompatibility renders androdioecy evolutionary stable (Vassiliadis et al, 2000). In this species, Saumitou-Laprade et al (2009) demonstrated the existence of two groups of self-incompatibility in hermaphrodites while males were compatible with all the hermaphrodites.

2.2 Functional adaptation to selfing and outcrossing in hermaphrodites

In flowering plants, physiological and morphological adaptations promoting outcrossing or selfing have been described. Many functional adaptations favoring cross-pollination are designed to promote pollen transfer. Floral design such as structure, odour, scent and nectar production are important components involved in plant/pollinator interactions (Barrett and Harder 1996). Reduction in flower size (petals) is often associated with the increase of self-fertilization. This is illustrated in figure 1 in the genus *Amsinckia* (Baroaginaceae). The outcrosser *A. furcata* displays large flowers whereas its close relative selfer *A. vernicosa* exhibits a reduced corolla (Schoen et al. 1997). Also, temporal separation of male and female function within an individual (protoginy and protandry) and spatial separation (herkogamy) are phenological adaptations to outcrossing. A widespread mechanism promoting outcrossing is the physiological inability for self-pollen to germinate on the stigma of the same flower, i.e. self-incompatibility, which is known to have evolved in many families (Barrett 1988). There are also functional adaptations to self-fertilization. A widespread floral adaptation to self-fertilization that has evolved in many botanic families has been described: cleistogamy (Lord 1981). It corresponds to the production of flowers that do not open, which implies obligate self-fertilization. Individuals generally produce both cleistogamous flowers and chasmogamous flowers (open flowers) and the proportion of each type has been found to be influenced by both genetic and environmental factors (Lord 1981).

2.3 The evolutionary transition from outcrossing to selfing or selfing as "an evolutionary dead end"

The evolution of self-fertilisation from outcrossing ancestors is a frequent transition in plant kingdom (Stebbins 1950). In this context, self-fertilising taxa have been considered to go extinct at higher rate than outcrossing taxon, which suggests that selfing lineages have short lifetimes. Takebayshi and Morell (2001) qualify the evolution towards selfing as "an evolutionary dead end". The loss of adaptive potential and reduced genetic variation have been proposed to account for the higher extinction of selfers but none of these hypotheses have been investigated empirically. As an illustrative example, Schoen et al. (1997)

studied the evolutionary history of mating system in the genus *Amsinckia* (Boraginaceae). The authors mapped mating system characters (i.e. population selfing rates) on the phylogeny of the genus (fig. 1). Assuming that the ancestral taxon was an outcrosser, the phylogeny reveals that selfing lineages have evolved four times in the genus, in an irreversible way.

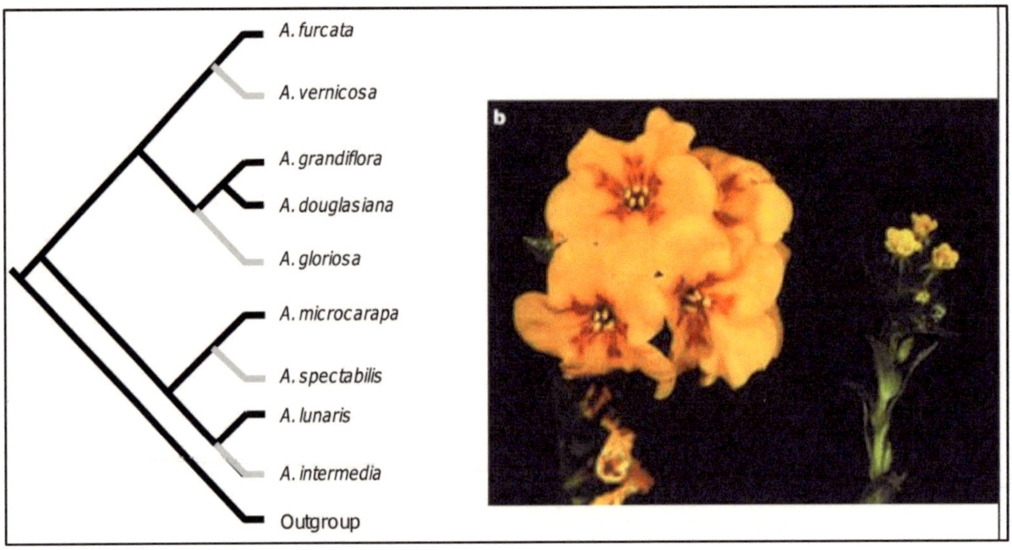

Fig. 1. Evolution of recurrent self-fertilization in the genus *Amsinckia* (Boraginaceae). The phylogenetic reconstruction is based on restriction site variation in the chloroplast genome (Schoen et al. 1997). In gray: branch giving rise to inbred lines, in black branch giving rise to cross-pollinated lines (the ancestor is supposed to cross-pollinated). Photos: left, the cross-pollinator *A. furcata* and right self-pollinating species *A. Vernicosa*. Courtesy of Daniel J. Schoen (McGill University, Canada).

In a recent study, Goldberg et al (2009) have demonstrated in the Solanaceae family that self-compatible species have a higher speciation rates than self-incompatible ones. However, extinction rate is much larger in self-compatible taxa resulting in a higher diversification rates for self-incompatible taxa. The apparent short-term advantages of self-compatible species are counterbalanced by strong species selection, thus favoring obligate outcrossing on the long-term. This study is unique and shows individual selection (or darwinian selection) may be insufficient to cature mating systems evolution in the phylogeny and that higher levels of selection may be at work.

2.4 The enigma of mixed selfing rates

Thanks to suitable techniques to measure plant mating systems, mating system biologists have created an important corpus of data. Two components have contributed to this development. The intensive use of neutral genetic markers (allozymes, microsatellites) have provided operational tools for mating system analysis (see Goodwillie et al 2005 for a recent compilation). In 1980's the distribution of selfing rates was considered to be bimodal with full outcrossers and full selfers (Schemske and Lande 1985) and conform to theoretical predictions. Admittedly, the few mixed selfers were considered to be transient states evolving towards full outcrossing or full selfing. The question of mixed selfing rates stimulated an important debate among mating system biologists to determine whether those selfing rates were transient states or stable states (Aide 1986; Waller, 1986).

An in-depth analysis and more complete data has revealed first that complete selfer are actually very rare. Second, that mixed selfing rates are relatively frequent, even if outcrossing rates exhibit a bimodal distribution (see Fig 2). Also genetic variations in selfing rates among close populations have been found (Bixby and Levin 1996; Cheptou et al. 2002) which suggests that mating systems respond quickly to selection. This implies that transient states could not be observed in natural populations in the case where disruptive selection operates. This intense debate in the 1990's has allowed the rise of new theoretical models discussing classical assumptions and demonstrating that the stability of mixed mating systems was possible.

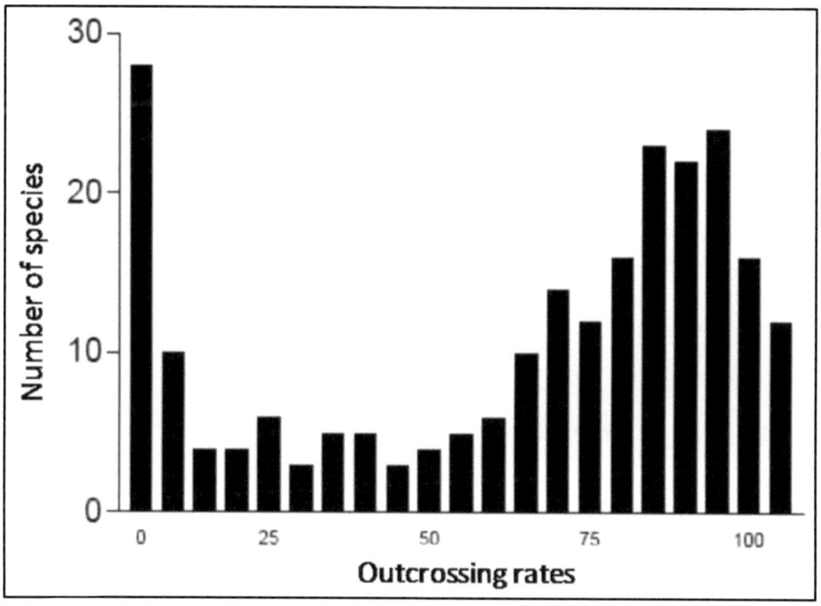

Fig. 2. Distribution of outcrosing rates in flowering plants (data from Vogler and Kalisz, 2001). Data courtesy of Susan Kalisz, University of Pittsburgh, USA.

3. Population genetics of self-fertilisation

3.1 Population genetics consequences of self-fertilization

Because self-fertilization defines gene transmission rules of individuals in a population, it has a predominant influence on major parameters of population genetics such as migration, recombination, selection and drift. As a consequence of mendelian segregation, heterozygotes produce half homozygotes each generation by self-fertilisation. At equilibrium, allelic diversity will be distributed among various classes of homozygotes under complete selfing, thus departing to the classical Hardy-Weinberg equilibrium under random mating. In a quantitative genetics perspective, selfing substantially affect the distribution of additive variance in a way that increases between-lines genetic variance and decreasing within line genetic variance as a consequence of the purity of the lines (Falconer, 1981). Self-fertilization will also modify the role of genetic drift in populations as consequence of the joint sampling of gametes. In diploid populations, male and female gametes are sampled independently under random mating, which results in an effective population size of twice the number of individuals. Because both female and male gametes are sampled together in individuals of a complete selfing population, the effective populations the population is only half the population size under random mating. The direct consequence is the more pronounced effect of drift in selfing populations resulting in a potential reduction of genetic diversity. Selfing can also affect genetic diversity by cancelling gene flow by pollen, which often disperse farther than seeds (Ghazoul, 2005), and thus increasing genetic drift. Biologists have analyzed the impact of selfing on genetic diversity and its distribution, thanks to the intensive use of neutral genetic markers in plants, or on the maintenance of additive genetic variance in quantitative traits. Using more than 250 plant species, Duminil et al (2009) showed that self-fertilisation increases among-population structure (Fst) and this effect is likely due to both its impact on gene flow (reduced pollen flow under selfing) and the reduced population sizes caused by inbreeding itself. Curiously, pollination modes, which are expected to modulate pollen gene flow, did not impact population structure.

Because selfing impacts the distribution of quantitative genetic variance of traits, one would expect the heritability of traits to be reduced under selfing, which could affect the evolutionary potential of populations. While early results have tended to support this trend (Clay and Levins, 1989), a rigorous analysis found no relationship between the partitioning of genetic variance within and among families and population selfing rates. Thus, empirical data does not support the idea that selfers respond less to selection than outcrossers.

3.2 The genetic basis of inbreeding depression

Inbreeding depression is defined has the reduction of fitness consecutive of one or several generations of inbreeding (*e.g.* selfing). This is a ubiquitous force in living organisms that has been documented in various organisms such as human, insects, birds, fish, crustaceans, ferns and higher plants (Cheptou and Donohue, 2011). Historically, the observations that inbred individuals are less fit than outbred ones have been documented more than 200 years ago by Thomas knight (1799) on vegetables. Darwin (1876) devoted an entire volume documenting the deleterious effects of inbreeding in 57 species. Interestingly, he anticipated a number of evolutionary trends, such as the relationship between inbreeding depression values and mating system of populations, which was to be confirmed by population genetics theory hundred years later. Beyond the empirical results reported in various organisms by empiricists, the rise of population genetics in the second half of the twenty century has allowed to develop a population genetics theory of inbreeding depression and to capture its genetic basis. The question of inbreeding depression can be formulated as follows: what are the genes characteristics required for fitness values to decrease as a consequence of increased homozygosity in a population? The answer can be characterized by considering a single locus encoding for any quantitative trait in a population and analyse the immediate consequence of inbreeding on fitness in this population. In a general way, we can write:

	AA	Aa	aa
Frequencies	D	H	R
Fitness values	*1*	*1-h s*	*1-s*

The mean population fitness can be easily deduced as $\overline{w_1} = 1 - s(h\,H + R)$. $\overline{w_1}$ can be compared to the mean population $\overline{w_2}$, the fitness after inbred mating, say one generation of selfing. After a bit of calculations, it can easily be shown that $\overline{w_2} = 1 - s(\frac{H}{2}(h+1) + R)$. We conclude that inbreeding depression occurs if $\overline{w_1} - \overline{w_2} = \frac{sH}{2}\left(\frac{1}{2} - h\right)$ is positive i.e. if $h < 0.5$. Two classical hypotheses satisfying this condition have been defined (Charlesworth and Willis, 2009). The partial dominance hypothesis ($0<h<1/2$) considers that partially recessive deleterious alleles ($s>0$) arise by recurrent mutations. The overdominance hypothesis considers that heterozygotes are fitter than both homozygotes ($h<0$). While overdominant alleles will be maintained at intermediate frequencies in populations as the result of balancing selection, deleterious alleles are typically expected to be at low frequencies as the result of mutation/selection balance. The relative importance of both hypotheses have been subject to intensive debate in the 1970's (Crow, 1993) but it is now admitted that the partial dominance hypothesis is the major source of inbreeding depression (Charlesworth and Willis, 2009). Empirical studies measuring mutation parameters have concluded that the rate of new deleterious mutation lies in the range of 0.1 to 1.0 per zygote per generation, and the reduction of fitness lies between 1 and 10% at homozygous state in metazoans (Schoen, 2005).

Whether natural populations should suffer from inbreeding depression or not depends on whether populations are regular inbreeders or not. While complete outcrossing is often viewed as a way to avoid inbreeding depression, the magnitude of inbreeding depression is in itself (measured as the difference in fitness in selfed and outcrossed offsprings) is not constant and vary with the inbreeding regime as a consequence of mutation selection balance in the populations. Importantly, the way the magnitude of inbreeding depression varies with the selfing regime under the partial dominance hypothesis and under the overdominance hypothesis is the exact opposite. If inbreeding depression is mainly due to overdominant alleles, inbreeding depression increases with selfing as a consequence the higher proportion of homozygote loci in inbred lines. On the contrary, if inbreeding depression is caused by deleterious alleles, inbreeding depression is expected to decrease with inbreeding regime. The reason is that regular inbreeding will expose recessive mutations to selection by producing homozygotes and thus lower the frequencies of deleterious alleles. This process known as the "purging process" has been central in population genetics studies analyzing inbreeding depression. Influential theoretical studies in the 1980-90's have modeled the expected relationship between inbreeding depression and selfing rates as a function of mutations parameters s, h (Lande and Shemske, 1985; Charlesworth et al, 1990). This has stimulated a large number of empirical studies attempting to measure inbreeding depression for various organisms with contrasted mating systems. The general trend in the data is mixed (see section 4). In a plant review, Husband and Schemske (1996) found a negative relationship between inbreeding depression and self-fertilisation, though weak, in accordance with expectations. However, a more complete compilation of data did were not able to find a significant decrease of inbreeding depression with selfing (Winn et al, 2011). Analysing specifically the possibility of purging in populations, Byers and Waller (1999) conclude that purging is an inconsistent forces in natural populations, thus casting doubt about the general applications of theoretical "purging" studies to natural populations.

3.3 Inferring mating system parameters in natural populations

How population genetics parameters vary with inbreeding and more specifically self-fertilization has been central in population genetics theory until its foundation (Malécot, 1948). The intensive use of polymorphic neutral markers (allozymes, microsatellites,...) in the last twenty years has allowed to estimate population selfing rates (and sometimes other parameters related to mating system) in natural populations. Classical methods use information related to homozygosity at one or several loci to infer selfing rates.

3.3.1 Inference from deviation to Hardy Weinberg equilibrium

The most popular method and probably the simplest one is based on the genotypic deviation to hardy-Weinberg equilibrium. Consider a simple locus with two alleles (A, freq. *p;* a freq. *1-p*). The genotypic frequencies can be written as follows:

	AA	Aa	aa
Hardy-Weinberg:	p^2	$2pq$	q^2
Deviation from H.W.:	$p^2 + pq\ F_{is}$	$2pq\ (1-F_{is})$	$q^2+pq\ F_{is}$

Under the assumption that heterozygotes deficiency is caused by selfing as the unique source of inbreeding (*e.g.* a large population of partial selfers), the equilibrium value F_{is} is related to selfing rate as $F_{is} = \frac{s}{2-s}$, where s is the population selfing rate. Thus, selfing rates can be easily inferred from genotyping a sample of individuals in a population. While this method is simple, F_{is} can be potentially inflated by other sources of inbreeding (biparental inbreeding) thus biasing upward the estimated selfing rates.

3.3.2 Inference from progeny array analysis

Another classical method to estimate selfing rates is based on the genotypic analysis of progenies. In plants, this can be easily achieved by sampling seeds on a mother plant. The genotypic composition of progeny results from medelian segregation under selfing and the random encounter of maternal alleles with alleles from the pollen pool under outcrossing. Thus, genotyping both the mother and the progeny allows to estimate selfing rates. Interestingly, this method allows inferring not only population estimates but also family estimates providing that sample sizes are adequate. Also, this method allows estimating additional parameters such the number of paternal parents in the outcrossed fraction *i.e.* if outcrossed progeny are full sibs or half sibs.

The MLTR program (Ritland, 1990, Ritland, 2002) is based on this method to infer selfing rates and additional parameters using maximum likelihood estimates. The procedures allows to distinguish the various sources of inbreeding: self-fertilisation and mating among related individuals (biparental inbreeding), through the comparison of multi-locus segregation and single-locus estimates. While this method provides relevant mating system parameters, its main drawback is that sample size must be large for good statistical inferences.

3.3.3 Inference from identity disequilibria

The two previous methods are based on the link between selfing and heterozygosity. While it is undoubtedly the most intuitive effect of selfing, it is important to recall that partial selfing not only creates heterozygote deficiencies but also creates correlations in heterozygosity among different loci, a process known as identity disequilibria (Weir & Cockerham 1973). Identity disequilibrium is the relative excess in doubly heterozygous genotypes (Weir & Cockerham 1973) for pairs of loci. The identity disequilibrium provides an additional source of information related to selfing available from neutral markers independent from heterozygotes deficiency. The main interest of this method is that, contrary to the previous method, identity disequilibria is relatively insensitive to the non-detection of heterozygotes (null alleles), which is a quite common scoring artifact in the use of molecular markers (e.g. microstaellites). David et al (2007) developed the Rmes software using identity disequilibria to estimate selfing rates. Interestingly, using several dataset, they showed that Fis tends to overestimate selfing rates as a consequence of putative scoring artifacts.

4. Plant mating system evolutionary theory: A long story

Darwin was the first of a long series of evolutionary botanists interested in mating system evolution (Darwin, 1876, 1877). At the heart of this approach was the central role of floral biology and pollination processes. As a consequence, the "pollination biology" tradition emphasizes on the role of ecological contexts. Population genetics, specifically the seminal work of Ronald Fisher, has changed the perspective by considering self-fertilisation as a gene transmission rule *i.e.* by emphasizing on intrinsic components of mating system biology, at the expense of ecological context in which mating system takes place. At the same time, population genetics has laid the foundation for a proper measure of fitness, which has paved the way for modeling evolutionary processes and capturing the role of various factors affecting the evolution of selfing.

4.1 Darwin' tradition versus Fisher's tradition

The first evolutionary principle for the selective advantage of selfing was proposed by Darwin (1876) who considered self-pollination as the mean of ensuring seed set either when outcrossing partners are absent or when pollinators are scarce. This has been referred to as the "reproductive assurance hypothesis" (Jain 1976). In the 1950's, Darwin's ideas have been largely popularized by the famous botanist Herbert Baker, who refined the arguments by proposing that such pollen limitation is likely to occur in species subject to recurrent colonization such as island colonizers, weeds or species on their limit range (Cheptou, 2011). Specifically, Baker (1955) proposed that: "With a self-compatible individual a single propagule is sufficient to start a sexually reproducing colony (after long distance dispersal), making its establishment much more likely than if the chance of the two self-incompatible yet cross-compatible individuals sufficiently close together spatially and temporally is required". Thus, reproductive assurance arguments focus on seed production under various ecological contexts *i.e.* on demographical properties of selfing.

While reproductive assurance is quite intuitive, Ronald Fisher highlighted another selective advantage of selfing based on gene transmission mechanisms (Fisher 1941) that defines the automatic avantage of selfing or the cost of outcrossing (Jain, 1976). He argued that genes favoring selfing (mating system modifiers) are automatically selected because they benefit from a 50% transmission advantage compared to "outcrossing" genes. This can be formally demonstrated using single locus model (see Annex 1). This can also be intuitively understood by considering that a selfer will transmit 2 copies of its genes in each of its selfed seeds and 1 copy by siring ovules by outcrossing in the population while an outcrosser will transmit only 1 copy in each of its seeds plus 1 copy by siring ovules by outcrossing in the population. It results in a 3:2 advantage for the selfer over the outcrosser (Figure 3). The cost of outcrossing is analogous to the cost of sex in gonochoric species (Maynard-Smith, 1978).

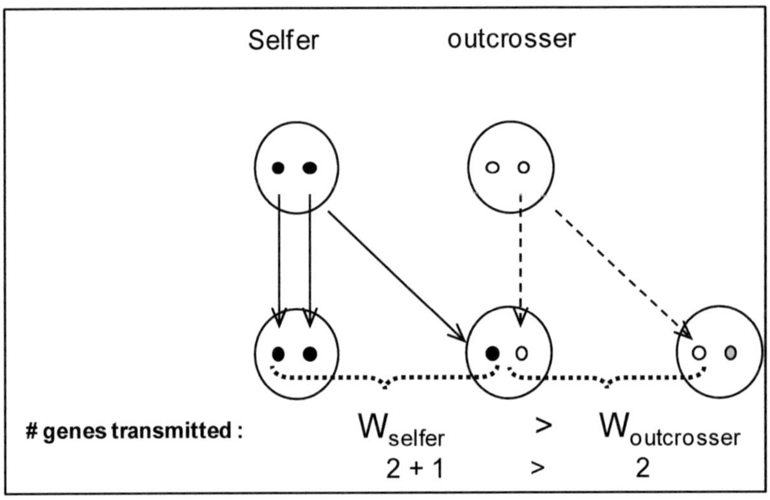

Fig. 3. Transmission pathways from parent to offspring are shown as arrows; solid arrows represent gene transmission to progeny by the parent capable of self-fertilization, while dashed arrows represent transmission pathways for the outcrossing parent. Fitness is expressed as the number of genes transmitted to the progeny via pollen and ovules. Assuming that the number of pollen grains produced is assumed to be large relative to the number of ovules (Bateman's principle), it results that a selfing genotype enjoy a 50% advantage in gene transmission relative to a outcrossing genotype.

While the two selective advantages of selfing described here are often presented without much details in the literature, it is important to note that they are not completely consistent with regards their underlying concept of fitness. The reproductive assurance argument is founded on the demographic advantage of selfing (seed production). Conversely, in the population genetic framework, the advantage of selfing is based on the number of genes transmitted. While the fitness metric defined by Fisher is relevant for evolutionary purpose, seed production is just a component of fitness but does not equate to the number of gene transmitted. In other words, reproductive assurance only considers the female component of fitness. Behind this discrepancy, pollination biologists have sometimes considered selfing advantage as the advantage of producing more seed (i.e. maternal contribution only) whereas fitness in the population genetics framework results from male and female contribution. In many studies (see for instance Klips and Snow, 1997), selfing advantages in Baker's arguments is based on a wrong fitness metric that does not match with the classical fitness metrics in mating system theory, which casts doubt about evolutionary inferences in such studies.

The major contribution of early population geneticists has been to define an unbiased metrics to measure the selective advantage of selfing, which has paved the way to build general evolutionary model for self-fertilisation.

4.2 Modeling the evolution of self-fertilization

Basically, the three general components: pollen limitation, the cost of outcrossing and inbreeding depression are the cornerstones of most theories for the evolution of self-fertilization. Lloyd (1979, 1992) was the first to model the evolution of self-fertilisation by including these three factors. Here, I present the general framework inspired from Lloyd work that allows deriving general results concerning factors affecting the evolution of selfing. For simplicity, I do not consider a diploid determinism for selfing but a phenotypic formalism, which, for our purpose, does not entail any changes in biological conclusions. Consider a large population of annual plants in which two phenotypes P_1 and P_2 differing for their mating strategies occur. Let be f_1 and f_2 be their respective frequencies. The fitness of each type can be derived as the sum of three components: selfed seeds, outcrossed seeds and pollen exported to outcross ovules in the population. The variables and the parameters of the model are described in Table 2.

Variables	# selfed ovules	# outcrossed ovules	# pollen grains (export)
Phenotype 1	y_1	x_1	p_1
Phénotype 2	y_2	x_2	p_2

Table 2. Variables used in model for the evolution of self-fertilisation (from Lloyd, 1979, Lloyd, 1992).

The deleterious effect of self-fertilisation is captured by the inbreeding depression parameter $\delta = 1 - \frac{w_{self}}{w_{out}}$ where w_{self} is the fitness of inbred progeny and w_{out} is the fitness of outbred progeny. The fitness component *via* pollen export requires to measure the relative succes of a pollen grain in the population. According to the notations, the pollen pool is $(f1p1 + f2p2)$ and the total number of ovules available for outcrossing is $(f1x1 + f2x2)$. Thus, the probablity for a pollen grain to fertilize an ovule is:

$$P = \frac{1}{(f1p1 + f2p2)} \cdot (f1x1 + f2x2) = \frac{\bar{x}}{\bar{p}}$$

Where $\bar{x}$ and $\bar{p}$ are the mean number of ovules per individuals devoted to outcrossing and the mean number of pollen grain exported repectively. Considering that inbreeding depression lowers the survival of selfed offrpsrings by a factor (1-δ), the fitness of the two phenotypes can be derived as:

$$W_1 = 2(1-\delta)y_1 + x_1 + p_1\left(\frac{\bar{x}}{\bar{p}}\right)$$

$$W_2 = 2(1-\delta)y_2 + x_2 + p_2\left(\frac{\bar{x}}{\bar{p}}\right)$$

At this stage, it is important to note that both fitness depend on each other *via* pollen export, which means that the selective advantage of selfing is frequency dependant. In a general way, phenotype 2 is favored over phenotype 1 if w_2-w_1>0, i.e :

$$2(1-\delta) > \underbrace{\left(\frac{x_1 - x_2}{y_2 - y_1}\right)}_{D_♀} + \underbrace{\left(\frac{p_1 - p_2}{y_2 - y_1}\right)}_{D_♂}\frac{\bar{x}}{\bar{p}}$$

Decomposing the inequality in such a way allows to analyse the different components of selection on selfing, namely: inbreeding depression (at the left-hand side), the functional relationship between the outcrossing x and selfing y ($D_♀$) and the functional relationship between pollen export p and selfing y ($D_♂$) at the right-hand side. According to Lloyd (1992), the two right-hand side components have a significant biological interpretation. First, the way the outcrossing fraction, x, varies with the increase of selfing ($D_♀$) defines the seed disounting and measures to what extent the outcrossing fraction and the selfing fraction compensate each other. In the hypothetical case where very few ovules are fertilised as the result of low pollination, increasing selfing may have no effect on reducing the outcrossing component ($D_♀ = 0$). On the opposite, if all the ovules are fertilised, the selfing fraction and outcrossing fraction counterbalance exactly each other ($D_♀$=1). The seed discounting parameter allows to estimate to what extent selfing increases seed production and thus provides a measure of reproductive assurance. Analogously, the pollen discounting parameter ($D_♂$) defines how increasing selfing affects pollen export. Fisher's automatic advantage (see figure 3) implicitely assumes that selfing strategy has no effect on pollen export *i.e.* there is no pollen discounting. As soon as pollen devoted to selfing decreases the amount of pollen export, the pollen discounting is positive thus reducing the 50% advantage of selfing described by Fisher (1941).

The model presented here allows to explore the role of parameters under various scenarios. The simplest case considers that every seed is either outcrossed or selfed, which leads to functional relationship: x=1-y. Also, if the number of pollen grains is large compared to the number of ovules (Bateman's principle) and thus pollen export is independant from selfing (*i.e.* p_1=p_2=$\bar{p}$), an inscrease in selfing rate is favored if:

$$\delta < \frac{1}{2}$$

In this context, inbreeding depression values lower than one half select for selfing whereas complete outcrossing is expected if inbreeding depression is higher than one half. I now use the same basic assumptions but I consider that only a fraction e of ovules devoted to outcrossing are actually fertilised because of reduced pollination activity. In this case, an inscrease in selfing rate is favored if $\delta < 1 - e/2$ *(e<1)*, which means that increase of selfing is easier under pollen limitation. This model has been very influential in mating system evolution and its conclusions are twofold. First, inbreeding depression values is sufficient to predict the direction of selection on selfing and second, it predicts that only complete selfing and complete outcrossing are evolutionary stable. As a consequence, mixed mating system cannot be considered as evolutionary stable in this framework.

4.3 The central role of inbreeding depression

The model exposed in 4.2 has stimulated much theoretical and empirical works on inbreeding depression. On theoretical perspective, much work has been devoted to the joint evolution of self-fertilisation and inbreeding depression. Given the genetic basis of inbreeding depression discussed in 3.2, population genetics models in the 1990's have analysed the evolution of selfing when inbreeding depression is free to evolve as a consequence of mutation/selection balance. These models have however shown that the conclusions with regards to the evolution of selfing were unchanged and the threshold of 0.5 still holds (Lande and Schemske, 1985). Interestingly, these models have allowed to predict the shape of inbreeding depression and genetic load as a function of the population selfing rates (see section 3). While the first population genetics models assumed a complete independence between fitness loci and selfing rate modifier loci, a few models have examined the joint evolution of loci affecting fitness and those affecting mating system. Holsinger (1988) was the first reveal that a more complex evolutionary dynamics evolves in this context. An important conclusion is that the precise 0.5 inbreeding depression threshold no longer holds. There are two reasons for this complex dynamics (Holsinger, 1991). First, there is a tendency for heterozygotes genotypes at one locus to be associated with heterozygotes at the other loci. Second, there is tendency for mating system modifier increasing diversity of fitness offspring to be associated with high fitness genotypes. This implies that an average inbreeding depression value over the whole population is not sufficient to predict the evolutionary outcome and that family inbreeding depression needs to be considered.

In line with the intense theoretical work on inbreeding depression, empiricists have produced a major contribution to inbreeding depression by providing an important corpus of data, using hermaphroditic plants but with contrasted selfing rates. These experiments are typically performed by crossing experimentally plants through outcrossing and selfing (hand pollination) and measure fitness traits on inbred and outbred progenies in order to estimate inbreeding depression. The motivation for such studies was twofold. First, in an evolutionary perspective, inbreeding depression values give information about its consistence with mating system in the populations in the context of the classical model presented in 4.2. Second, the relationship between inbreeding depression values and selfing rates among populations or among species allow inferring the genetic basis of inbreeding depression (overdominance hypothesis *versus* partial dominance hypothesis). In particular the possibility of purging has been at the heart of many studies.

Figure 4 represents the compilation of nearly all inbreeding depression values in plants reported in the literature. This figure shows that the relationship with selfing is not clear-cut and the high variation of inbreeding depression values for a given selfing rate suggests that other factors affect inbreeding depression values.

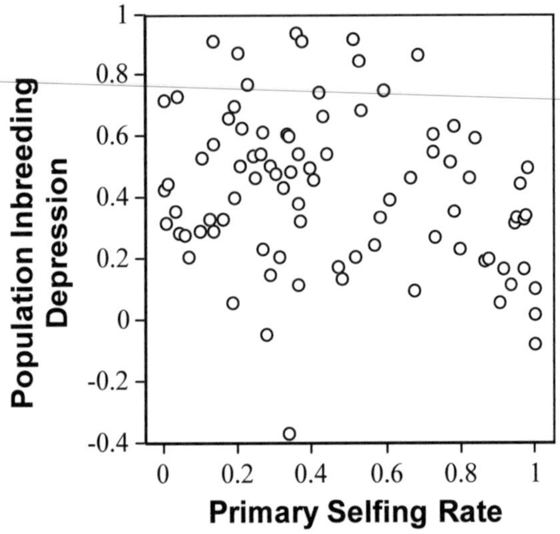

Fig. 4. Relationships between experimental inbreeding depression and primary selfng rates (estimated from microsatellites markers) in 87 plant populations (data taken from Winn et al, 2011).

5. Towards a synthesis between ecology and population genetics

Population genetics theory in the 1980's and 90's has provided a general framework for analyzing the evolution of selfing rates. While the ecological tradition of mating system is ancient and influential, the approach has been rather empirical with little mathematical formalism. Thanks to fruitful confrontation between theory and data, the last twenty years have given rise to a more integrated view, taking into account genetic and ecological factors affecting mating system. Below, I give three directions where the synthesis has been particularly fruitful.

5.1 Pollination biology and gene transmission rules

Pollination biologists have for a long time described with many details the patterns of pollen transfer among plants. Pollen transfer involves various such as wind, water of animals. Insect pollination has been by far the most studied pollination processes. Specific plant adaptations in animal-pollinated plants have been well-studied. A well studied example is heterostyly where two (or three) floral designs differing in the spatial arrangement of female (pistil) and male (stamen) organs. This is typically viewed as an adaptation to the morphogy of insects implying that one type can only mate with the other in the population (Barrett, 2002). In such a system, the pollen removed on plant type 1 sticks in a specific place on insect body and is deposited on the pistil of plant type 2 (and vice versa). In light of Fisher's argument described in fig 3, pollination biology of species may imply that pollen export is dependent on mating strategies which may affect the automatic advantage of selfing. The example of cleistogamous plants widespread in flowering plant (Lord, 1981) provides a comprehensive view of the problem. In such a plant producing both open (chasmogamous) and close (cleistogamous) flowers, selfing rates is mediated by cleistogamy. Because cleistogamy prevents any possibility of pollen export, increasing selfing rates implies a direct reduction of pollen export *i.e.* complete pollen discounting (see 4.2). It results that the automatic advantage of selfing no longer works in cleistogamous plants. This example highlights that patterns of pollen export are fundamental to capture Fisher's advantage of selfing. This pollination consideration has led to a new class of evolutionary models analyzing the role of pollen discounting in the selection of selfing. In particular, Holsinger (1991) proposed a very elegant and intuitive evolutionary model, the "mass-action model" based on simple pollination mechanism. In his model, selfing rates simply results from the relative portion of self-pollen and outcross pollen deposited on the stigma *i.e.*

$$s = \frac{\#\,self\ pollen}{\#\,self\ pollen + \#\,outcross\ pollen}$$

Thus, changing the selfing strategy for a plant consists in modifying the exportation of pollen. A fully outcrossing population is a population where all the genotypes export their pollen whereas a full selfing population is a population where all the genotypes do not export their pollen. Because the model assumes compensation between pollen exported and pollen devoted to selfing, pollen discounting is at the heart of the model. The evolutionary dynamics is interesting and allows the evolution of stable mixed selfing on a large range of parameters, which the classical model did not predict. The reasons for such dynamics are quite intuitive. In a full outcrossing population, it is easy to demonstrate that keeping a small portion of its pollen on its own stigmas may be advantageous, if pollen export is costly (pollen lost during travel). In full selfing population (no pollen export), it is advantageous to export a small fraction of its pollen to avoid self-pollen competition on the stigma. These two lines of arguments indicate that evolutionary stable mixed selfing is possible under mass action assumption. More generally, the discussion around the notion of pollen discounting has allowed to reinterpret the automatic advantage of selfing in the context of pollination biology. It allowed to aknowledge that the 50% advantage, often taken for granted in early studies is not a fixed parameter but a consequence floral biology such as the pollen/ovule ratio (Cruden, 1977), itself subject to natural selection.

5.2 The ecology of inbreeding depression

If inbreeding depression experiments have been motivated by theory, an unexpected experimental issue has provided a new direction for the role of inbreeding depression in mating system evolution. Though measuring inbreeding depression may seem simple at first sight, it has revealed that environmental conditions in which plants grow were determinant. While the theory did not reject this idea a priori, the fact that empiricists had no conceptual framework to interpret their results lead some authors to consider it a nuisance or a side effect that should avoided (Barrett and Harder, 1996). Yet, this phenomenon has been identifed by early biologists. In 1876, Darwin wrote:

> *The result was in several cases (but not so invariably as might have been expected) that the crossed plants did not exceed in height the self-fertilized in nearly so great a degree as when grown in pairs in the pots. Thus with the plants Digitalis, which competed together in pots, the crossed were to the self-fertilized in height as 100 to 70; whilst those which were grown separately were only as 100 to 85. Nearly the same result was observed with Brassica. With Nicotiana the crossed were to the self-fertilized in height, when grown extremely crowded*

together in pots, as 100 to 54; when grown much less crowded in pots as 100 to 66, and when grown in the open ground, so as to be subjected to but little competition, as 100 to 72.

Darwin's observation of the environmental dependence of inbreeding depression has since been reported in diverse organisms in experimental studies (Keller & Waller, 2002; Armbruster & Reed, 2005). Interestingly, direct estimates in natural populations based on the change in inbreeding coefficient during plant life cycle have also revealed that inbreeding depression may vary until four times from one year to the other (Dole and Ritland, 1993). These results ask the question of whether environment-dependant change the evolutionary dynamics of self-fertilisation or if it can be considered as a side-effect. Cheptou and Donohue (2011) have discussed this problem and conclude that environment-dependant inbreeding depression is worth to be considered in an ecological and evolutionary perspective. In this context, the relevant question is to identify the pattern of environment-inbreeding depression. Beyond the simple stress dependence of inbreeding depression (Armbruster and Reed, 2005) it is important to capture what causes the environment-dependence. For instance Cheptou and Schoen (2003) have shown experimentally in the genus *Amsinckia* that the identity of competitors was fundamental to predict inbreeding depression in density-regulated populations. By manipulating the proportion inbred and outbred individuals in competing stands (at constant density), Cheptou and Schoen (2003) reported that the magnitude of inbreeding depression is highly sensitive to the inbred/outbred proportions (frequency-dependence). Since this proportion is the direct consequences of population selfing rates in natural populations, the authors conclude that taking into account the environmental feedback caused selfing rates is crucial to capture the selective effect of inbreeding depression on selfing (see also Cheptou and Dieckmann, 2002). Interestingly, taking into account this effect gives a consistent picture for the evolution of selfing in *Amsinckia douglasiana* (Cheptou and Schoen, 2003).

In a theoretical model, Cheptou and Mathias (2001) consider a simple ecological scenario where inbreeding depression vary from year to year because of random environmental variation ($Pr(\delta=\delta_1)=p$, $Pr(\delta=\delta_2)=1-p$). In the context of inbreeding depression/automatic advantage of selfing (see 4.2), the authors demonstrated the evolutionary stability of mixed selfing rates, and found that the evolutionary stable selfing rate is:

$$s^* = \frac{1+2\delta_2(p-1)-2\delta_1 p}{(1-p)\delta_1 - 2\delta_1\delta_2 + \delta_2 p}$$

So far, the evolutionary models including environment-dependant inbreeding depression have been phenomenological models (see however Porcher et al, 2009), with little interest to the genetic basis of environment dependant inbreeding depression. Ronce et al (2009) analyzed a quantitive genetics model where local adaptation occurs. Assuming several environments where optimal phenotypes differ, they showed that inbreeding depression can vary as a function of the distance between the population mean breeding value for a trait under stabilizing selection and the optimal phenotype. In Ronce et al (2009) model, inbreeding depression is a function of the genetic variance for a trait under selection and the strength of stabilizing selection. An important result is that inbreeding depression is always lower when the population is less adapted to its environment compared with well-adapted populations.

More generally, the rise of environment-dependant inbreeding depression has changed the perspective regarding the evolution of selfing. Experimental studies analyzing inbreeding depression in 2010's now take into account environment in their designs. This phenomenon challenges the applicability of mutation–selection balance models where the deleterious effects is fixed. To what extent is inbreeding depression caused by unconditionally deleterious alleles or by loci under balancing selection? This problematic revitalizes the question of the genetic basis of inbreeding depression and the maintenance of diversity for alleles contributing to inbreeding depression in natural populations.

5.3 Mating system and metapopulation dynamics

In Baker's view, the importance of space and spatio-temporal heterogeneity is at the heart of the evolution of selfing. Indeed, by considering colonization processes as determinants in pollination services, Baker points out that not only population processes are relevant in mating system evolution but also among population processes *i.e.* metapopulation processes. Curiously, most of mating system models have assumed evolutionary processes in a single population in a stable environment until recently. There are two reasons for this fact. First, population genetic theory has implicitly adhered to the classical assumption of a unique population. Second, the fitness metric considered in Baker's arguments does not match with classical mating system theory (see 4.1), which does facilitate the mix between the two traditions.

Two recent models (Pannell and Barrett, 1998; Dornier et al., 2008) have however provided a mathematical formalization for Baker's law where pollination is related to the number of mates. Hence, their assumption is close to Baker's first argument: 'with a self-compatible individual a single propagule is sufficient to start a sexually reproducing colony, making its establishment much more likely than if the chance growth of two self-incompatible yet cross compatible individuals sufficiently close together spatially and temporally is required'. While Pannell and Barrett (1998) analysed the advantage of colonization by a single individual allowed by selfing, Dornier et al. (2008) considered a metapopulation model with an explicit Allee effect function and random extinction of patches. Interestingly, Dornier et al. (2008) derived analytically a metapopulation viability criterion that is dependent on the selfing rate. Whereas full out-crossers can form a viable metapopulation, only partial selfers and full selfers are able to recover from very low density at the regional scale. Both models demonstrate the intuitive conclusion that when the number of colonizers is low, selfing is favored. Dornier et al (2008) revealed an interesting feature of the model. Because inbreeding depression affect demography, two colonizers for an out-crosser may have the same probability of arriving in a colonizing area than one colonizer for a selfer. For the same set of parameters, the number of colonizers can increase with outcrossing rate and favor outcrossing, so that mating strategy tends to self-reinforce itself. By disentangling forces at work in Baker's law, these models have demonstrated than selfing is not necessarily selected in colonizing organism, which echoes with empirical data (Cheptou, 2011). Another class of models analyzing the joint evolution of selfing and dispersal traits under stochastic pollination has revealed that the classical colonizer syndrome which assumes that disperser are also selfers is far from being the rule and that the opposite syndrome emerges from metapopulation dynamics (Cheptou and Massol, 2009).

6. Conclusion

In this review, I attempted to present a general overview of the field by focusing on the major trends of the discipline. Mating system biologists have studied plant and its evolution for more than two hundred years. As such, plant mating system has fed one of the most important fields of research in evolutionary biology and it is still very active. Interestingly, this field has many connections with major theme of research in population genetics (role of mutations), pollination biology and even genetic breeding program in agronomy. The important corpus of data coupled with intensive theory allowed us to analyse processes with a large perspective. Plant mating system studies provide an integrative analysis of the processes articulating genetical components in ecological context. To a certain extent, one could say that the domain has reached maturity. Also, the long story of mating system biology has revealed that mating system is a complex trait that cannot so easily summarize by a simple metric such as selfing rate. In this respect, mating system may be consider as a syndrome of traits and considering the joint evolution of integrated traits is an interesting perspective to follow. Finally, enlarging mating system concepts to spatially heterogeneous landscapes is undoubtedly a fruitful approach. Incidentally, it could help to understand how plants will react to changes in pollination environment in the context of pollinator decline.

7. Appendix 1

The automatic advantage of selfing (Fisher, 1941).

Let us consider a biallelic locus coding for selfing rates. For simplicity, consider the allele *A* encoding for self-fertilisation and the allele *a* encoding for outcrossing. Assuming that *A* is dominant over *a*, this leads to three genotypes (two phenotypes):

	AA	Aa	aa
Selfing rates	100%	100%	0%

(f_1, f_2, f_3 are the genotypes frequencies of AA, Aa, aa respecively and $p = f_1 + \frac{f_2}{2}$ and $q = f_3 + \frac{f_2}{2}$ are the allelic frequencies of A and a respectively).

Let us now consider the genotypic frequencies at the next generations (denoted by f_i'):

$$f_1' = f_1 + \frac{f_2}{4}$$

$$f_2' = \frac{f_2}{4} + f_3 . p$$

$$f_3' = \frac{f_2}{4} + f_3 . q$$

And thus allelic frequencies at the next generation:

$$p' = f_1' + \frac{f_2'}{2} = f_1 + \frac{f_2}{4} + \frac{f_2}{4} + \frac{f_3}{2} p$$

Variation in the frequency of allele a is :

$$p' - p = f_1 + \frac{f_2}{2} + \frac{f_3}{2}\,p - \left(f_1 + \frac{f_2}{2}\right)$$

$$p' - p = \frac{f_3}{2}\,p$$

Because allelic and genotypic frequencies are by definition positive (or null), this shows allele A encoding for self-fertilisation increases in frequency until fixation, thus demonstrating the automatic advantage of selfing.

8. References

Aide, M. T. (1986). "The influence of wind and animal pollination on variation in outcrossing rates." Evolution 40(2): 434-435.

Armbruster, P. and D. Reed (2005). "Inbreeding depression in benign an stressfull environments." Heredity 95: 235-242.

Baker, H. G. (1955). "Self-compatibility and establishment after "long distance" dispersal." Evolution: 347-348.

Barrett, S. C. H. (1988). The evolution, maintenance, and loss of self-incompatibility systems. Plant reproduction ecology, Oxford University Press: 98-124.

Barrett, S. C. H. and L. D. Harder (1996). "Ecology and evolution of plant mating system." TREE 11(2): 73-79.

Barrett, S.C.H. (2002). The evolution of plant sexual diversity. Nature Reviews Genetics 3: 274–284

Barrett S.C.H. (ed.) (2008). Major Evolutionary Transitions in Flowering Plant Reproduction. University of Chicago Press, Chicago, USA

Bawa, K. S. (1980). "Evolution of dioecy in flowering plants." Annual Review of Ecology and Systematics 11: 15-39.

Bixby, P. J. and D. A. Levin (1996). "Response to selection on autogamy in phlox." Evolution 50(2): 892-899.

Byers, D. L. and D. M. Waller (1999). "Do plant populations purge their genetic load? Effects of population size and mating system history on inbreeding depression." Annual Review of Ecology and Systematics 30: 479-513.

Clay, K. and D. A. Levins (1989). "Quantitative variation in Phlox: comparison of selfing and outcrossing species. ." American Journal of Botany 76: 577-589.

Charlesworth, D. 1984 Androdioecy and the evolution of dioecy Biological Journal of the Linnean Society Vol 22 (4), pp 333–348.

Charlesworth, D., M. T. Morgan, et al. (1990). "Inbreeding depression, genetic load, and the evolution of outcrossing rates in a multilocus system with no linkage." Evolution 44(6): 1469-89.

Charlesworth, D. and J. H. Willis (2009). "The genetics of inbreeding depression." Nature reviews genetics 10: 783-796.

Charnov, E. L., J. Maynard-Smith, et al. (1976). "Why be an hermaphrodite?" Nature 263(5573): 125-126.

Cheptou, P. O. and A. Mathias (2001). "Can varying inbreeding depression select for intermediairy selfing rates?" The American Naturalist 157(4): 361-373.

Cheptou, P. O., J. Lepart, et al. (2002). "Mating system variation along a successional gradient in the allogamous and colonizing plant Crepis sancta (Asteraceae)." Journal of Evolutionary Biology 15(5): 753-762.

Cheptou, P. O. and U. Dieckmann (2002). "The evolution of self-fertilization in density-regulated populations." Proceedings of the Royal Society of London (B) 269: 1177-1186.

Cheptou, P. O. and D. J. Schoen (2003). "Frequency-dependent inbreeding depression in *Amsinckia*." The American Naturalist 162(6): 744-753.

Cheptou, P.-O. and K. Donohue (2011). "Environment-dependant inbreeding depression : its ecological and evolutionary significance." New phytologist 189: 395-407.

Cheptou, P.-O. 2011 Clarifying Baker's law. Annals of Botany (early view).

Cheptou, P. O. and F. Massol (2009). "Pollination Fluctuations Drive Evolutionary Syndromes Linking Dispersal and Mating System." American Naturalist 174(1): 46-55.

Crow, J. F. (1993). Mutation, mean fitness, and genetic load, Oxford Suvey in Evolutionary Biology. 9: 3-42.

Cruden, R.W. 1977. Pollen–ovule ratios – conservative indicator of breeding systems in flowering

plants. Evolution, 31: 32–46.

David, P., B. Pujol, et al. (2007). "Reliable selfing rate estimates from imperfect population genetic data." Molecular Ecology 16: 2474-2487.

Darwin, C. (1862). The various contrivances by which orchids are fertilized. London, John Murray.

Darwin, C. R. (1876). The effects of cross and self fertilization in the vegetable kingdom. London, Murray.

Darwin, C. R. (1877). The different forms of flower on plants of the same species. London, Murray.

Dole, J. and K. Ritland (1993). "Inbreeding depression in two Mimulus taxa measured by multigenerationnal changes in inbreeding coefficient." Evolution 47(2): 361-373.

Dornier, A., F. Munoz, et al. (2008). "Allee Effect and Self-Fertilization in hermaphrodites: Reproductive Assurance in a Structured Metapopulation." Evolution 62(10): 2558-2569.

Duminil, J., O. J. Hardy, et al. (2009). "Plant traits correlated with generation time directly affect inbreeding depression and mating system and indirectly genetic structure." Bmc Evolutionary Biology 9.

Falconer, D. S. (1981). Introduction to quantitative genetics. Essex, England, Longman Scientific & Technical.

Fisher, R. A. (1941). "Average excess and average effect of a gene substitution." Ann. Eugen. 11: 53-63.

Ghazoul, J. (2005). "Pollen and seed dispersal and dispersed plants." Biological Review 80: 1-31.

Goldberg, E. E., J. R. Kohn, R. Lande, K. A. Robertson, S. A. Smith, and B. Igic. 2010. Species selection maintains self-incompatibility. Science 330:459-460

Goodwillie, C. et al. (2005) The evolutionary enigma of mixed mating systems in plants: occurrence, theoretical explanations, and empirical evidence. Annu. Rev. Ecol. Evol. Syst. 36, 47–79.

Gouyon P.H. & Couvet D. 1988. A conflict amongst the sexes, Females and Hermaphrodites.in The evolution of sex. S.C. Stearns ed. Birkhauser verlag. pp. 245-261.

Husband, B. and D. W. Schemske (1996). "Evolution of the magnitude and timing of inbreeding depression in plants." Evolution 50(1): 54-70.

Holsinger, K. E. (1988). "The evolution of self-fertilization in plants : lessons from populations genetics." Acta oecologica 9(1): 95-102.

Holsinger, K. E. (1991). "Inbreeding depression and the evolution of plant mating systems." TREE 6(10): 307-308.

Holsinger, K. E. (1991). "Mass action models of plant mating systems : the evolutionary stability of mixed mating systems." Am. Nat. 138(3): 606-622.

Jain, S. K. (1976). "The evolution of inbreeding in plants." Ann. Rev. Ecol. Syst. 7: 469-495.

Keller, L. F. and D. M. waller (2002). "Inbreeding effects in wild populations." Trends in Ecology and Evolution 17(5): 230-241.

Jarne, P. and D. Charlesworth (1993). "The evolution of the selfing rate in functionally hermaphrodite plants and animals." Ann. Rev. Ecol. Syst 24: 441-466.

Keller, L. F. and D. M. waller (2002). "Inbreeding effects in wild populations." Trends in Ecology and Evolution 17(5): 230-241.

Klips RA, Snow AA. 1997. Delayed autonomous self-pollination in Hibiscuslaevis (Malvaceae). American Journal of Botany 84: 48–53.

Knight, T. (1799). "Experiments on the fecundation of vegetables." Philosophical Transcations of the Royal Society of London 89: 195-204.

Lande, R. and D. W. Schemske (1985). "The evolution of self fertilization and inbreeding depression in plants. I. Genetic models." Evolution 39(1): 24-40.

Lord, E. M. (1981). "Cleistogamy: a tool for the study of floral morphogenesis, function and evolution." The Botanical Review 47(4): 421-449.

Lloyd, D. G. (1979). "Some reproductive factors affecting the selection of self-fertilization in plants." American Naturalist 113(1): 67-79.

Lloyd, D. G. (1992). "Self and cross fertilization in plants. 2-The selection of self fertilization." Int. J. Plant Sci. 153(3): 370-380.

Malécot, G., 1948 Les mathématiques de l'hérédité. Masson, Paris.

Maynard Smith, J. (1978). The evolution of sex. London New-York Melbourne, Cambridge University Press.

Pannell, J. R. and C. H. Barrett (1998). "Bakers'law: reproductive assurance in a metapopulation." Evolution 52(3): 657-668.

Porcher, E., J. K. Kelly, et al. (2009). "The genetic consequences of fluctuating inbreeding depression and the evolution of plant selfing rates." Journal of Evolutionary Biology 22(4): 708-717.

Richard, A. J. (1986). Plant Breeding Systems. George Allen & Unwin, London. 529 p.

Ritland, K. (1990). "A series of FORTRAN computer programs for estimating plant mating systems." Journal of heredity 81: 235-237.

Ritland, K. (2002). "Extensions of models for the estimation of mating systems using n independent loci." Heredity 88: 221-228.

Ronce, O., F. H. Shaw, et al. (2009). "Is inbreeding depression lower in maladapted populations? A quantitative genetics model" Evolution 63(7): 1807-1819.

Saumitou-Laprade, P. Vernet, P, Vassiliadis, C. Hoareau, Y. de Magny, G. Dommée, B. and Lepart, J. 2009 A Self-Incompatibility System Explains High Male Frequencies in an Androdioecious Plant Vol. 327 no. 5973 pp. 1648-1650 Science.

Schemske, D. W. and R. Lande (1985). "The evolution of self fertilization and inbreeding depression in plants : empirical observations." Evolution 39(1): 41-52.

Schoen, D. J., M. O. Johnston, et al. (1997). "Evolutionay history of the mating system in *Amsinckia* (Boraginaceae)." Evolution 51(4): 1090-1099.

Schoen, D.J. 2005. Spontaneous deleterious mutation in wild plant species with contrasting mating systems. *Evolution*, 59: 2370-2377.

Stebbins, G. L. (1950). Variation and evolution in plants. New York, USA., Columbia University Press.

Takebayashi, N. and L. F. Delph (2000). "An association between a floral trait and inbreeding depression." Evolution 54(3): 840-846.

Uyenoyama, M. K., K. E. Holsinger, et al. (1993). Ecological and genetic factors directing the evolution of self fertilization. O. S. i. e. biology. 9: 327-381.

Vassiliadis, C. Valero, M. Saumitou-Laprade, P and Godelle, B. 2000 A model for the evolution of high frequencies of males in an androdioecious plant based on a cross-compatibility advantage of males. Heredity 85, 413

Vogler, D. W. and S. Kalisz (2001). "Sex among the flowers: the distribution of plant mating systems." Evolution 55(1): 202-204.

Waller, D. M. (1986). "Is there a disruptive selection for self-fertilization?" American Naturalist 128(3): 421-426.

Weir, B. S. and C. C. Cockerham (1973). "Mixed self and random mating at two loci." Genetical Research 21: 247–262.

Winn, A.A., Elle, E., Kalisz, S., Cheptou, P.-O., Eckert,C.G., Goodwillie, C. Johnston,M.O., Moeller, D.A., Ree, R.H., Sargent, R.D. and Vallejo-Marın, M. 2011 Analysis of inbreeding depression in mixed mating plants provides evidence for selective interference and stable mixed mating *Evolution* (early view).

Yampolsky, C. and H. Yampolsky (1922). "Distribution of sex forms in the phanerogamic flora." Bibl. Genet. 3: 1-62.

3

Population Genetics of the "*Aeromonas hydrophila* Species Complex"

Mª Carmen Fusté, Maribel Farfán, David Miñana-Galbis,
Vicenta Albarral, Ariadna Sanglas and José Gaspar Lorén
*Department of Health Microbiology and Parasitology, Faculty of Pharmacy,
University of Barcelona, Barcelona,
Spain*

1. Introduction

Population genetics studies the genetic variability of individuals in a population based on the allele frequencies at several genes or loci and tries to explain this variability in terms of mutation, selection or genetic recombination. The statistical analysis of these frequencies allows models of evolution to be established, which will help us to understand and predict the past and present gene flow in the population (Maynard-Smith, 1991). For the most part population genetics has been designed for diploid organisms with sexual reproduction. In the words of Bruce Levin, "the genetic theory of adaptive evolution was developed by sexually reproducing eukaryotes, for sexually reproducing eukaryotes" (Levin & Bergstrom, 2000). As a consequence, before being applied to prokaryotes, population genetics needs to be adapted.

In theory the haploid nature of bacteria should simplify their analysis, since dominance or over-dominance is not an issue and the genotype can usually be deduced directly from the phenotype. However, central to classical population genetics are infinite population size, random mating, and free recombination. Consequently, as expressed by Maynard-Smith, "the alleles present at one locus are independent of those at other loci. Changes in the frequency of an allele at one locus, therefore, are independent of what is happening elsewhere in the genome: each locus can be treated individually" (Maynard-Smith, 1995). It is true that the size of bacterial populations can be practically infinite but recombination occurs extremely rarely so that changes affecting one locus can lead to the modification of others. In the succinct words of Maynard-Smith, "the genome should be treated as an inter-related whole, and not as a set of independently changing genes". The crux of the problem is knowing the exact level of recombination in bacterial populations, since "it is considerably more challenging to elaborate a theory for a population with little recombination than for one with no recombination, or a lot" (Maynard-Smith, 1995). In bacterial population genetics, sometimes we detect a degree of recombination that is too high for a pure phylogenetic approach, but too low for assessing a random interchange.

Stronger evidence for restricted recombination comes from measurements of linkage disequilibrium: that is, the tendency for particular alleles at different loci to co-occur

(Maynard-Smith et al., 1993; Haubold et al., 1998). Linkage disequilibrium (and the too-frequent occurrence of a particular combination of alleles, which is a manifestation of such disequilibrium) shows that recombination is restricted, but not absent. The determination of the relative importance of mutation in comparison with recombination is central to bacterial population genetics (Feil et al., 1999). Previous studies have demonstrated a wide variety of situations among bacterial species ranging from the clonal diversification of *Salmonella* (Selander et al., 1990) or *Escherichia coli* (Orskov et al., 1990), which are mainly due to mutation, to the frequent recombination found in *Neisseria gonorrhoeae* (O'Rourke & Stevens, 1993) or *Helicobacter pylori* (Salaun et al., 1998). Most of the population studies done with bacterial species suggest that recombination occurs in nature, and indeed may be highly important in generating variation, but that it is infrequent compared to mutation. Consequently, bacterial populations consist largely of independent clonal lineages.

The development of protein electrophoresis was a breakthrough for the study of bacterial population genetics. A pioneer in the field, Milkman (1973) used the methodology to study whether electrophoretic variation is selective or neutral. As described by Selander et al., Multilocus Enzyme Electrophoresis (MLEE) "has long been a standard method in eukaryotic population genetics and systematics" before it was applied "for studying the genetic diversity and structure in natural populations of bacteria. This research established basic population frameworks for the analysis of variation in serotypes and other phenotypic characters and has provided extensive data for systematics and useful marker systems for epidemiology" (Selander et al., 1986).

In 1998, Maiden et al. introduced Multilocus Sequence Typing (MLST), an extension of MLEE based on nucleotide sequencing that is able to determine higher levels of discrimination (more alleles per locus). In MLST "alleles are identified directly from the nucleotide sequences of internal fragments of genes rather than by comparing the electrophoretic mobilities of the enzymes they encode" (Maiden et al., 1998). In addition, this method is fully portable between laboratories and data can be stored in a single multilocus sequence database accessible via the internet (http://www.mlst.net). This approach has given "a new dimension to the elucidation of genomic relatedness at the inter- and intraspecific level by sequence analysis of housekeeping genes subject to stabilising selection. This technique has been mainly used in epidemiology, but it offers the opportunity to incorporate the insights available from population genetics and phylogenetic approaches into bacterial systematics" (Stackebrandt et al., 2002; Pérez-Losada et al., 2005; Robinson et al., 2010).

The results obtained using MLST indicate that despite the high diversity observed in bacteria, it is possible to recognize clusters with a lower degree of variation. The number of sequence types (STs) obtained is less than expected if we consider the product of the individual allelic frequencies. Nevertheless, most of the strains belong to one or a few allelic profiles, whereas most of the STs are represented by one or few strains. In addition, most STs cluster in clonal complexes constituted by closely related genotypes. Typically, each clonal complex consists of a predominant ST and a varied group of less common STs, which have different alleles only in one or two loci (Feil et al., 2004). These differences could correspond to initial stages of clonal divergence from an ancestral genotype that was the origin of the clone (Vogel et al., 2010; Willems, 2010).

2. The genus *Aeromonas*

The genus *Aeromonas* Stanier 1943 belongs to the family *Aeromonadaceae* within the class *Gammaproteobacteria* (Martin-Carnahan & Joseph, 2005). Aeromonads are autochthonous inhabitants of aquatic environments including chlorinated and polluted waters, although they can also be isolated from a wide variety of environmental and clinical sources. They cause infections in vertebrates and invertebrates, such as frogs, birds, various fish species and domestic animals. In recent years, some authors have considered *Aeromonas* as an emergent pathogen in humans, producing intestinal and extraintestinal diseases. Aeromonads are facultative anaerobic chemoorganotrophs capable of anaerobic nitrate respiration and dissimilatory metal reduction (Martin-Carnahan & Joseph, 2005).

The interest in the taxonomy of the genus *Aeromonas* has increased markedly in recent years (Janda & Abbott, 2010), and its classification, with 25 species currently recognized, remains challenging. Novel species are continuously being described, strains and species described so far are being rearranged, and DNA-DNA hybridization studies have observed discrepancies (Janda & Abbott, 2010). Historically, the genus *Aeromonas* has been divided into two groups: nonmotile, psychrophilic species, best represented by *A. salmonicida*, which are generally associated with fish diseases and motile mesophilic species associated with human diseases, including *A. hydrophila*, *A. veronii* and *A. caviae* (Martin-Carnahan & Joseph, 2005). More species have since been described and genealogies have to be adapted accordingly, although this is not always straightforward.

Bacterial species are formally defined as a group of strains that share several phenotypical characteristics and show values of DNA-DNA hybridization ≥ 70% and a 16S rRNA sequence similarity ≥ 97% with their close relatives (Stackebrandt et al., 2002). Indeed, there are hardly any examples in which strains with divergence in the 16S rRNA sequence ≤ 97% are defined as one species (Roselló-Mora & Amann, 2001). In *Aeromonas* 16S rRNA gene sequences are highly similar, being identical in some close related species such as *A. salmonicida*, *A. bestiarum*, *A. popoffii* and *A. piscicola*, which hampers their utility in defining species in this genus (Figueras et al., 2000; Beaz-Hidalgo et al., 2009).

Several attempts have been made to generate phylogenies using DNA gene sequences to reconstruct the correct genealogical ties among species in *Aeromonas* (Küpfer et al., 2006; Saavedra et al., 2006; Miñana-Galbis et al., 2009), but the genes chosen for this purpose are not always suitable and do not give congruent phylogenies (Farfán et al., 2010; Silver et al., 2011). Recently, two papers presenting MLST schemes for *Aeromonas* have been published (Martínez-Murcia et al., 2011; Martino et al., 2011) and there is an online MLST database of the genus *Aeromonas*, managed by Keith Jolley and curated by Barbara Cardazzo (http://pubmlst.org/aeromonas). All this accumulated data should help to establish a reliable clustering of the *Aeromonas* species and elucidate their exact boundaries.

Finally, the availability of complete genomes of different species is also useful in this task, but unfortunately in the case of *Aeromonas* only three genomes have been completed, one corresponding to the type strain of *A. hydrophila* subsp. *hydrophila* ATCC 7966 isolated from a tin of milk (Seshadri et al., 2006), the second to a fish pathogen, the strain A449 of *A. salmonicida* subsp. *salmonicida* (Reith et al., 2008) and the third to *A. veronii* isolated from an aquaculture pond sediment (Li et al., 2011). The information given by the genomes of *A. hydrophila* and *A. salmonicida* indicate that while they are of identical size (4,7Mb) and share multiple housekeeping and virulence genes, *A. salmonicida* has acquired several mobile genetic elements, and undergone genome rearrangements and loss of genes in the process of adapting to a specific host. The genome of *A. veronii* is smaller (4,3Mb) and contains fewer virulence genes than the others.

3. "*Aeromonas hydrophila* species complex"

An example of the taxonomic complexity of the genus *Aeromonas* is the difficulty in discriminating between the phenotypically and genetically closely related species belonging to the "*Aeromonas hydrophila* species complex" (AHC), which includes: *A. hydrophila,* composed by three subspecies: A. *hydrophila* subsp. *hydrophila, A. hydrophila* subsp. *ranae* and *A. hydrophila* subsp. *dhakensis, A. bestiarum, A. popoffii* and *A. salmonicida,* divided in five subspecies: *A. salmonicida* subsp. *salmonicida, A. salmonicida* subsp. *masoucida, A. salmonicida* subsp. *achromogenes, A. salmonicida* subsp. *pectinolytica* and *A. salmonicida* subsp. *smithia* (Miñana-Galbis et al., 2002; Martin-Carnahan & Joseph, 2005). Recently, two additional species have been described in this group, *A. aquariorum* and *A. piscicola* (Martínez-Murcia et al., 2008; Beaz-Hidalgo et al., 2009). Members of the AHC were first described as strains producing the enzymes elastase, lecitinase or stapholysin (Abbott et al., 2003). They are genetically closely related and share multiple phenotypic characteristics, which makes discrimination among the species included in this group extremely difficult (Miñana-Galbis et al., 2002).

Several approaches have been used to discriminate among the AHC species: Amplified Fragment Length Polymorphisms (AFLP) (Huys et al., 1997), fluorescent AFLP (FAFLP) (Huys et al., 2002), MLEE (Miñana-Galbis et al., 2004), Random Amplified Polymorphic DNA (RAPD) and MALDI-TOF MS analysis (Martínez-Murcia et al., 2008). Although the results obtained with these methods have been useful for the taxonomy and phylogeny of the AHC, providing a hypothesis for the genealogy of strains and detailing their patterns of descent and degree of genetic variation accumulated over time, only the MLEE study has been used to elucidate their population genetic structure.

Previous studies based on the sequence analysis of several housekeeping genes have demonstrated that the AHC is not monophyletic (Soler et al., 2004; Küpfer et al., 2006; Saavedra et al., 2006; Nhung et al., 2007; Beaz-Hidalgo et al., 2009; Miñana-Galbis et al., 2009). Nevertheless, controversially, other studies have shown the monophylia of this group (Martínez-Murcia et al., 2005; Farfán et al., 2010). This conflict could be due to the incongruence of phylogenies derived from distinct gene sequence analysis.

In order to establish the population structure and divergence of the species included in this group of *Aeromonas* we studied a set of strains representative of the AHC, in which we analyzed the nucleotide sequences (total or partial) of 6 housekeeping genes: *cpn*60 (555 bp), *dna*J (891 bp), *gyr*B (1089 bp), *mdh* (936 bp), *rec*A (1065 bp), *rpo*D (843 bp), giving a total fragment length of 5379 bp.

4. Phylogenetic analysis

The relationships among the analyzed *Aeromonas* isolates are represented as a genealogical tree (Fig. 1). The tree reveals that the AHC splits into three main clusters separated by a mean genetic distance of 0.071 (Table 1). The *A. salmonicida* cluster, although comprising five subspecies, constitutes a homogeneous clade with the lowest mean genetic distance of 0.016 (Table 1). The closest relative to *A. salmonicida, A. bestiarum,* has a different population structure. Rather than being a single group, it is divided in three clades, one constituted by the great majority of the *A. bestiarum* strains, a second corresponding to *A. popoffii* and the third including some *A. bestiarum* strains together with isolates of *A. piscicola.* The mean genetic distance of the *A. bestiarum* cluster is higher than in *A. salmonicida* 0.029 (Table 1). The *A. hydrophila* group, which exhibits the highest genetic distance 0.037 (Table 1), clearly separates in two clades, one including the *A. hydrophila* subsp. *hydrophila* and *A. hydrophila* subsp. *ranae* and the second constituted by *A. hydrophila* subsp. *dhakensis* and *A. aquariorum.* The presence of different clades in some of these species poses questions about the clade-species relationships.

	TN93	**Standard error**
All sequences	0.0717	0.0024
A. bestiarum	0.0286	0.0014
A. bestiarum (clade 1)	0.0157	0.0009
A. bestiarum (clade 2)	0.0084	0.0008
A. bestiarum (clade 3)	0.0100	0.0008
A. hydrophila	0.0370	0.0016
A. hydrophila (clade 1)	0.0219	0.0010
A. hydrophila (clade 2)	0.0158	0.0012
A. salmonicida	0.0163	0.0009

Table 1. Mean genetic distances for all sequences and clusters calculated using the Tamura Nei (1993) distance. Standard error estimates were obtained by the bootstrap method with 500 replicates.

	TN93	**Standard error**
A. bestiarum vs. *A. salmonicida*	0.0655	0.0033
A. bestiarum vs. *A. hydrophila*	0.1042	0.0043
A. hydrophila vs. *A. salmonicida*	0.1101	0.0049
A. bestiarum (clade 1) vs. *A. bestiarum* (clade 2)	0.0507	0.0027
A. bestiarum (clade 1) vs. *A. bestiarum* (clade 3)	0.0279	0.0021
A. bestiarum (clade 2) vs. *A. bestiarum* (clade 3)	0.0526	0.0031
A. hydrophila (clade 1) vs. *A. hydrophila* (clade 2)	0.0558	0.0030

Table 2. Mean genetic distances among different clusters obtained using the Tamura Nei (1993) distance. Standard error estimates were obtained by the bootstrap method with 500 replicates.

Estimation of distance frequency within and between clusters from multilocus sequence data provides interesting insights into the population structure of these groups. The frequency distribution of the pairwise genetic distances clearly identifies the AHC species phylogenetic structure (Fig. 2). Within the strains of the *A. bestiarum* group (Fig. 2A), the plot shows three peaks with distance values ranging from 0 to 0.063. The lowest values correspond to pairwise comparisons among isolates within clades (1, 2 and 3) and the highest to those between clades. Distances between groups allowed a clear separation of *A.*

bestiarum from the other species groups. When we plotted the pairwise distance distribution within the *A. hydrophila* group (Fig. 2B) two peaks were shown and again the lowest values are those within the clades and the highest between the clades (0-0.062). *A. hydrophila* is clearly separated from *A. salmonicida* and *A. bestiarum* despite the overlap in the graph (Fig. 2B), which is a consequence of the similar distance values between *A. hydrophila* and *A. salmonicida* (0.110) and *A. hydrophila* and *A. bestiarum* (0.104). Otherwise, species boundaries are objectively defined in the phylogenetic tree (Fig. 1). In the *A. salmonicida* group, the within distance distribution (0-0.030) appears as a single peak, as does the interspecies distance.

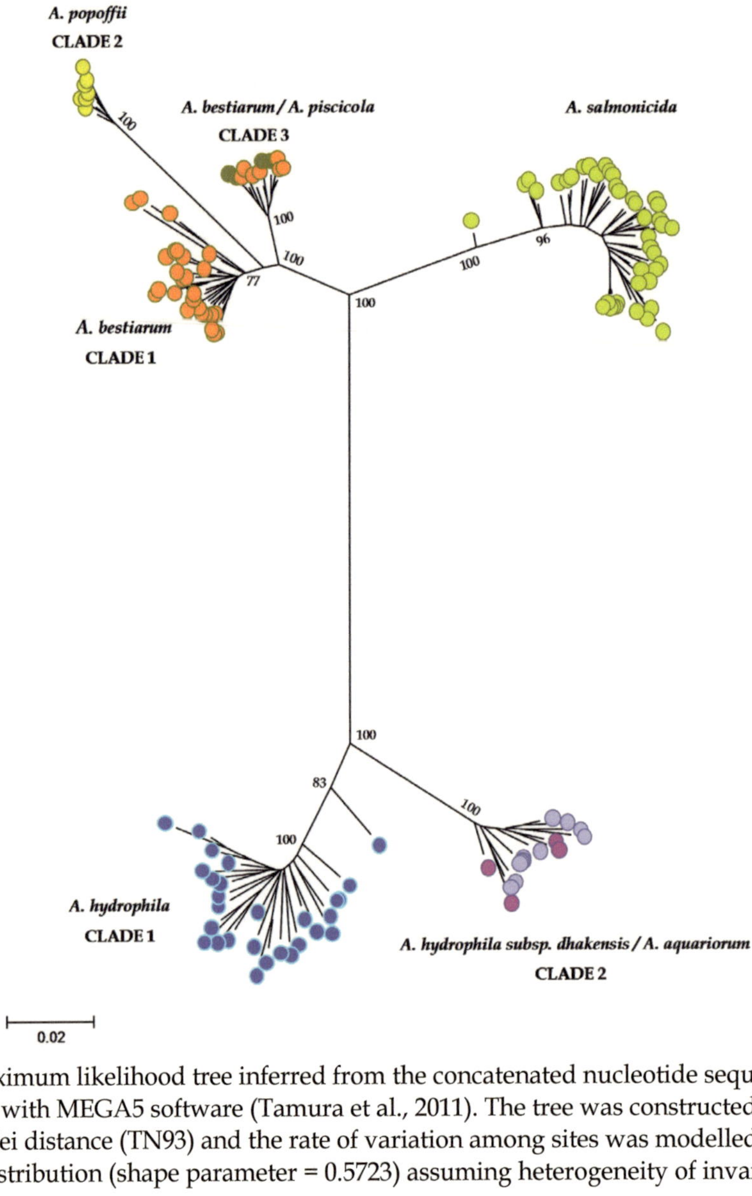

Fig. 1. Maximum likelihood tree inferred from the concatenated nucleotide sequences generated with MEGA5 software (Tamura et al., 2011). The tree was constructed using the Tamura Nei distance (TN93) and the rate of variation among sites was modelled with a gamma distribution (shape parameter = 0.5723) assuming heterogeneity of invariant sites

(best model for the data). Numbers at the branch nodes represent bootstrap values (500 replicates). The scale bar indicates the number of nucleotide substitutions per site. The GenBank/EMBL/DDBJ accession numbers of the nucleotide sequences used in this study are EU306796-EU306797, EU306804-EU306806, EU306814-EU306820, EU306822-EU306824, EU306826-EU306829, EU741625, EU741635-EU741636, EU741642, FJ936120, FJ936135, GU062399, JN711508-JN711610 (*cpn60* gene); FJ936122, FJ936136, JN215529-JN215534, JN711611-JN711731 (*dnaJ* gene); FJ936137, JN215535, JN711732-JN711858 (*gyrB* gene); HM163293-HM163294, HM163305-HM163307, HM163312-HM163318, JN660159-JN660273 (*mdh* gene); JN660274-JN660400 (*recA* gene) and EF465509-EF465510, FJ936132, FJ936138, JN215536-JN215541, JN712315-JN712433 (*rpoD* gene).

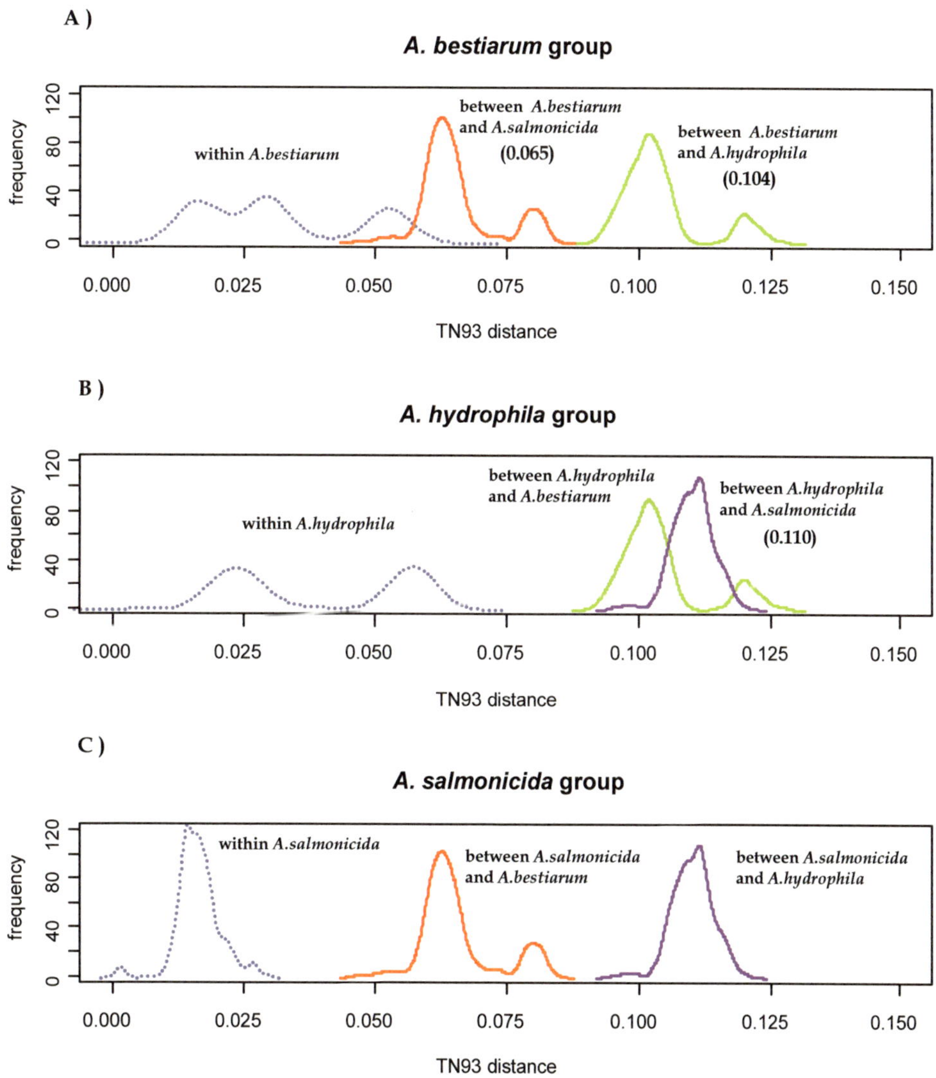

Fig. 2. Distribution of TN93 distances within and between clusters determined by pairwise comparisons. Mean distances are indicated within brackets.

Although to our knowledge there is no function that could be used to define a level of divergence for distinguishing species, it seems clear that, in bacteria, there is always an exponential relationship between interspecies recombination and sequence divergence (Roberts & Cohan, 1993; Zawadzki et al., 1995; Vulic et al., 1997). Values of divergence among clades (Table 2) seem to correspond to those of a genetically isolated biological species. The lowest value corresponds to *A. bestiarum* clade 3, indicating that its isolates are undergoing speciation, but species boundaries are not as well-defined as in the other clades.

5. Linkage disequilibrium and population structure

Linkage equilibrium is characterized by the statistical independence of alleles at all loci. A common method used in bacterial population genetics to quantify the degree of linkage between a set of loci in MLSA data is to use the index of association (I_A) (Brown et al., 1980; Maynard-Smith et al., 1993). This index compares the ratio of variance calculated from the pairwise distribution of allele mismatches in the data (V_O) and the ratio expected under a null hypothesis of linkage equilibrium (V_E). In this case

$$E(V_O) = \sum h_j (1-h_j),$$

where h_j is an unbiased estimator of the population genetic diversity equivalent to heterozygosis in diploid organisms (Table 4). The index of association (I_A) originally used by Brown et al. (1980) is computed as

$$I_A = V_O / V_E - 1,$$

which would give a value of zero if there is no association between loci (Maynard-Smith et al., 1993). Values of this index significantly different from zero reflect strong linkage disequilibrium (lower rates of recombination). The value of I_A depends on the number of loci analyzed. Haubold & Hudson (2000) subsequently proposed a standardized index of association ($I_A{}^S$) defined as

$$I_A{}^S = (1/l-1)\, I_A,$$

where l is the number of loci studied. This index has the advantage of being comparable between studies as long as it can be assumed that the neutral mutation parameter $\theta = 2Ne\mu$ is constant (Hudson, 1994). Two methods are commonly used for determining whether the computed I_A represents a significant deviation from linkage equilibrium ($I_A \sim 0$): resampling from randomized data sets using Monte Carlo simulations or using the parametric method described by Haubold et al. (1998). Both methods are perfectly good alternatives.

The genetic structure of the AHC, which has been previously determined using enzyme electrophoresis (MLEE), has revealed a clear clonal structure with strong linkage disequilibrium among 15 different protein loci (Miñana-Galbis et al., 2004). Additionally, this study demonstrated the usefulness of MLEE for separating the strains belonging to *A. bestiarum* and *A. salmonicida*, which are almost indistinguishable by phenotypic characteristics and 16S rRNA sequence analysis and present borderline DNA-DNA homology values.

In a multilocus sequence analysis (using six housekeeping genes) of a new set of AHC strains in which we included representatives of *A. piscicola* and *A. aquariorum*, we obtained

I_A^S values different from 0 in all cases, indicating the absence of recombination and again revealing strong linkage disequilibrium when considering both the total population and the different groups of species (Table 5). This is in spite of the high number of alleles per locus and polymorphic sites (Table 3) and huge genetic diversity (Table 4). Values of V_O, V_E, I_A^S and the 5% critical values as determined by the Monte Carlo process (L_{MC}) and from the parametric approach (L_{para}) of Haubold et al. (1998) are shown in Table 5.

Gene	Number of alleles	Number of polymorphic sites	π ± s.e.**
cpn60	95	144	0.075 ± 0.009
dnaJ	102	237	0.082 ± 0.007
gyrB	108	266	0.063 ± 0.005
*mdh**	113	225	0.059 ± 0.009
*recA**	106	282	0.071 ± 0.009
rpoD	110	212	0.090 ± 0.010

* full-length sequence gene; ** nucleotide diversity (π) ± standard error (s.e.)
Calculated by using MEGA5 software (Tamura et al., 2011).

Table 3. Sequence variation at six loci. Standard error estimates were obtained by the bootstrap method with 500 replicates.

	STs	h_j*						H ± s.e.**
		cpn60	*dnaJ*	*gyrB*	*mdh*	*recA*	*rpoD*	
All STs	127	0.9931	0.9959	0.9966	0.9978	0.9945	0.9973	0.9959 ± 0.0007
A. bestiarum	44	0.9704	0.9863	0.9863	0.9905	0.9852	0.9873	0.9843 ± 0.0029
A. hydrophila	42	0.9930	0.9884	0.9954	1.0000	0.9930	0.9930	0.9938 ± 0.0015
A. salmonicida	41	0.9744	0.9902	0.9878	0.9890	0.9707	0.9951	0.9846 ± 0.0039

* genetic diversity at individual loci (h_j); ** mean genetic diversity (H) ± standard error (s.e.)
$h_j = (n/n\text{-}1)\sum p_{ij}^2$, where p_{ij} is the frequency of the *i*th allele at the *j*th locus and *n* the number of loci.
Data were calculated by using R statistical software (R Development Core Team, 2010).

Table 4. Genetic diversity (h) at six loci for all STs and major species sets.

	V_O	V_E	I_A^S	L_{para}	L_{MC}	P_{MC}
All STs	0.0635	0.0248	0.3131	0.0253	0.0255	$< 1.00 \times 10^{-04}$
A. bestiarum	0.2314	0.0924	0.3010	0.0986	0.1001	$< 1.00 \times 10^{-04}$
A. hydrophila	0.1382	0.0369	0.5495	0.0395	0.0405	$< 1.00 \times 10^{-04}$
A. salmonicida	0.1916	0.0908	0.2222	0.0978	0.0988	$< 1.00 \times 10^{-04}$

For the meaning of acronyms, see text. The L_{MC} and P_{MC} results were obtained from 10000 resamplings. Data were calculated by using R statistical software except for L_{para}, which was determined with the LIAN 3.5 program (Haubold & Hudson, 2000).

Table 5. Multilocus linkage disequilibrium analysis of the AHC.

During the last years, with the availability of the first DNA sequence data of individual genes, evidence of recombination at the molecular level has accumulated for *Aeromonas* in genes such as *dnaJ*, *gyrB* and *recA* (Silver et al., 2011). Incongruence between trees reconstructed from individual genes appeared as further proof of recombination at the gene level. Nevertheless, multilocus analysis with gene sequences also revealed a clear clonal structure in this bacterial group (Table 5). The question is that although bacteria are capable of accumulating gene fragments from other bacterial species or mutations, the recombinant segments are not long enough to break the clonal structure of the population. While the absence of linkage (I_A^S ~ 0) is difficult to explain without assuming high levels of recombination, linkage disequilibrium does not exclude the presence of significant levels of recombination (Touchon et al., 2009).

In our study we have also determined the presence of recombinant fragments in the *recA* (in four *A. bestiarum* strains) and *dnaJ* genes (five strains, 2 *A. bestiarum*, 2 *A. hydrophila* and 2 *A. salmonicida*). However, although these strains cluster separately when the corresponding tree is constructed, revealing the different origin of the gene fragments, they group together with the other strains when a concatenated tree is generated. This confirms that recombination is not sufficient to break the genetic cohesion of this group.

6. Gene flow and divergence

The existence of barriers to gene flow such as geographical separation, ecological adaptation or the accumulation of genetic differences ultimately leads to distinct lineages. These processes are usually more complicated in prokaryotes, since the boundaries of their species are sometimes distorted by gene transfer between divergent organisms. In addition, the mechanisms that can contribute to the cohesion of groups are very different in bacteria. We have determined the divergence among the different AHC clades using the nucleotide fixation index, N_{ST} (Nei & Kumar, 2000). The use of the N_{ST} as a measure of population differentiation under certain circumstances has been criticized (Jost, 2008), but it is still used for describing the average amount of such differentiation observed from multiple locus data (Ryman & Leimar, 2009). In our study, the determination of the N_{ST} values indicated a high level of interclade genetic differentiation (N_{ST} = 0.8025). On average, most of the 80% of the total variance of nucleotide diversity was attributable to genetic differentiation among clades, whereas about 20% was found within populations. High levels of diversification were also found among most of the AHC groups of species (Table 6), with values always higher than 0.7 except in the case of *A. bestiarum* clade 3 / *A. bestiarum* clade 1 (N_{ST} = 0.5) and *A. hydrophila* clade 2 / *A. hydrophila* clade 1 (N_{ST} = 0.6). The clear divergence between the different clades described suggests they form coherent groups in which the phenomenon of recombination, if present, fails to break this consistency.

In bacterial populations it seems reasonable to equate the effect of lateral gene transfer (LTG) from other species with the product *Nm* (effective population size x migration rate) determined from N_{ST}. Indeed, assuming the limitations of the Wright island model (Wright, 1940), the value of N_{ST} at the equilibrium ($1/(2Nm+1)$) allows *Nm* to be calculated. The values obtained for all AHC clades (N_{ST} = 0.8, *Nm* ~ 0.13) again suggest that gene flow (in this case, the lateral gene transfer) is insufficient to counteract their genetic differentiation.

The McDonald-Kreitman Test (MKT, McDonald & Kreitman, 1991) was applied to our data sets to detect signs of selection (Table 7). Under neutrality, the ratio of nonsynonymous-to-synonymous fixed substitutions (between species) should be the same as the ratio of nonsynonymous-to-synonymous polymorphism (within species). We observed a high level of fixed replacements between most species studied. In all comparisons the ratio of nonsynonymous-to-synonymous substitutions was higher for fixed differences than for polymorphisms. This result agrees with the presence of mutations under positive selection spreading quickly through a population. These changes do not contribute to polymorphism but have a cumulative effect on divergence and the fixed NS/S is consequently greater than polymorphic NS/S (Egea et al., 2008). Two of the McDonald-Kreitman tests were not significant, *A. bestiarum* versus *A. salmonicida* and *A. piscicola* (*A. bestiarum* clade 3) versus the other strains of the *A. bestiarum* group.

	***A. best* clade 1**	***A. best* clade 2**	***A. best* clade 3**	***A. hyd* clade 1**	***A. hyd* clade 2**	***A. salm***
A. bestiarum clade 1	---	0.1703	0.4532	0.1366	0.1068	0.1907
A. bestiarum clade 2	0.7460	---	0.1174	0.0863	0.0683	0.1051
A. bestiarum clade 3	0.5245	0.8099	---	0.1077	0.0833	0.1480
A. hydrophila clade 1	0.7854	0.8529	0.8228	---	0.1264	0.1264
A. hydrophila clade 2	0.8240	0.8798	0.8571	0.6428	---	0.0993
A. salmonicida	0.7239	0.8264	0.7716	0.7982	0.8343	---

Calculated using DnaSP v5.10 software (Librado & Rozas, 2009).

Table 6. Pairwise estimates of population differentiation, N_{ST} (lower-left) and gene flow, *Nm* (upper-right).

	Fixed		*Polymorphic*		*NI*	*P*
	S	NS	S	NS		
A. bestiarum vs. *A. hydrophila*	83	26	1235	88	0.227	0.000000 ***
A. bestiarum vs. *A. salmonicida*	57	7	964	77	0.650	0.325391 ns
A. hydrophila vs. *A. salmonicida*	118	36	1141	86	0.247	0.000000 ***
A. bestiarum (clades 1 and 3) vs. *A. bestiarum* (clade 2)	88	15	596	43	0.423	0.015757 *
A. bestiarum (clade 1 and 2) vs. *A. bestiarum* (clade 3)	21	3	659	48	0.510	0.402179 ns
A. hydrophila (clade 1) vs. *A. hydrophila* (clade 2)	56	16	803	48	0.209	0.000009 ***

Acronyms are for synonymous substitutions (S); nonsynonymous substitutions (NS); neutrality index (*NI*); *P*-value from Fisher's exact test (*P*). * $0.01<P<0.05$; ** $0.001<P<0.01$; *** $P<0.001$; not significant (ns). Calculated using DnaSP v5.10 software (Librado & Rozas, 2009).

Table 7. McDonald-Kreitman Test for molecular evidence of selection.

7. Conclusions

Developments in gene sequence analysis have greatly enhanced the study of bacterial population genetics. Gene-wide approaches to mapping bacterial diversity, which have already proved effective for gaining fresh insight into bacterial evolution, have the potential to reveal the phenotypic basis of genetic diversity in the AHC and to investigate the dynamics of this complex bacterial community. The general objective of the work described in this chapter has been to evaluate the suitability of combining population genetics and phylogenetic approaches for the delineation of bacterial species in the AHC, considered by many specialists a taxonomically tangled group.

The results obtained from the linkage disequilibrium analysis and sequence divergence show that the AHC is composed of four robust groups that basically correspond with the phenotypically described species *A. hydrophila*, *A. bestiarum*, *A. popofii* and *A. salmonicida*. The average divergence between these clusters seems to exclude a significant influence of recombination in the genetic structure of this bacterial group and therefore they are valid taxonomic units, despite the extensive variability within some of them. Phenotypic characteristics lead to the differentiation of five *A. salmonicida* subspecies, but the lack of a consistent signal in our multilocus sequence analysis only allowed the possible differentiation of *A. salmonicida* subsp. *pectinolytica*. Similarly, it is impossible to differentiate between *A. hydrophila* subsp. *hydrophila* and *A. hydrophila* subsp. *ranae*. These results are in agreement with those obtained in a previous study with isolates belonging to the *A. veronii* Group, in which the authors failed to achieve the differentiation of biovars within these *Aeromonas* species (Silver et al., 2011). Nevertheless, *A. hydrophila* subsp. *dhakensis* strains, which cluster together with *A. aquariorum* isolates, exhibited the divergence levels of a biological species and hence deserve full species status. Consequently, the *A. aquariorum* isolates should be reclassified. Finally, in the *A. bestiarum* group we distinguished a clade (clade 3) that includes *A. piscicola* isolates as well as several strains probably misclassified as *A. bestiarum*. This clade seems to constitute an incipient new species with low values of differentiation and species boundaries less well defined than in *A. bestiarum* (clade 1) or *A. popofii* (clade 2).

It has been frequently postulated that in bacterial populations, lateral gene transfer is so common that it precludes the existence of true biological species. One of the aims of this study has been to verify if this hypothesis is applicable to our AHC data. Three lines of evidence suggest the contrary. First of all, using the Tamura Nei model, which best fits our data, we found considerable interspecific nucleotide diversity, suggesting a high degree of divergence that hampers recombination among AHC species. Secondly, the linkage disequilibrium analysis of six loci reveals a strong disequilibrium with $I_A{}^S$ values, suggesting little or null influence of recombination in the genetic structure of AHC species. Thirdly, the N_{ST} values obtained reflect a high degree of differentiation between clades. In short, the genetic structure of the AHC appears to confirm that the entities phenotypically described as species form cohesive groups in which genetic recombination plays a limited role in reducing genetic variation and can be defined as biological species.

Like other authors (Lan & Reeves, 2001; Vinuesa et al., 2005), we agree that a combination of phylogenetic and population genetic studies is currently the best theoretical and practical approach to delineate species as natural and discrete lineages in the bacterial world.

8. Acknowledgments

We are very grateful to Katri Berg (University of Helsinki, Finland), Margarita Gomila (Universitat de les Illes Balears, Mallorca, Spain) and Carmen Gallegos (Hospital Sant Llàtzer, Mallorca, Spain) for kindly providing some of the strains used in this study. This research was supported by the project CGL-2008-03281/BOS from the Ministerio de Educación y Ciencia, Spain.

9. References

Abbott, L.S.; Cheung, W.K.W. & Janda, M.J. (2003). The genus *Aeromonas*: Biochemical characteristics, atypical reactions, and phenotypic identification schemes. *Journal of Clinical Microbiology*, Vol. 41, No. 6, pp. 2348-2357.

Beaz-Hidalgo, R.; Alperi, A.; Figueras, M.J. & Romalde, J.L. (2009). *Aeromonas piscicola* sp. nov., isolated from diseased fish. *Systematic and Applied Microbiology,* Vol. 32, No. 7, pp. 471-479.

Brown, A.D.; Feldman, M.W. & Nevo, E. (1980). Multilocus structure of natural populations of *Hordeum spontaneum*. *Genetics,* Vol. 96, No. 2, pp. 523-536.

Egea, R.; Casillas, S. & Barbadilla, A. (2008). Standard and generalized McDonald-Kreitman test: a website to detect selection by comparing different classes of DNA sites. *Nucleic Acids Research,* Vol. 36, No. 2, pp. W157-W162.

Farfán, M.; Miñana-Galbis, D.; Garreta, A.; Lorén, J.G. & Fusté, M.C. (2010). Malate dehydrogenase: a useful phylogenetic marker for the genus *Aeromonas*. *Systematic and Applied Microbiology,* Vol. 33, No. 8, pp. 427-435.

Feil, E.J.; Maiden, M.C.J.; Achtman, M. & Spratt, B.G. (1999). The relative contributions of recombination and mutation to the divergence of clones of *Neisseria meningitidis*. *Molecular Biology and Evolution,* Vol. 16, No. 11, pp. 1496-1502.

Feil, E.J.; LI, B.C.; Aanensen, D.M.; Hanage, W.P. & Spratt, B.G. (2004). eBURST: Inferring patterns of evolutionary descent among clusters of related bacterial genotypes from multilocus typing data. *Journal of Bacteriology,* Vol. 186, No. 5, pp. 1518-1530.

Figueras, M.J.; Soler, L.; Chacón, M.R.; Guarro, J. & Martínez-Murcia, A.J. (2000). Extended method for discrimination of *Aeromonas* spp. by 16S rDNA RFLP analysis. *International Journal of Systematic and Evolutionary Microbiology,* Vol. 50, No. 6, pp. 2069-2073.

Janda, J.M. & Abbott, S. (2010). The genus *Aeromonas:* taxonomy, pathogenicity, and infection. *Clinical Microbiology Reviews,* Vol. 23, No. 1, pp. 35-73.

Jost, L. (2008). G_{ST} and its relatives do not measure differentiation. *Molecular Evolution,* Vol. 17, No. 18, pp. 4015-4026.

Haubold, B.; Travisano, M.; Rainey, P.B. & Hudson, R.R. (1998). Detecting linkage disequilibrium in bacterial populations. *Genetics,* Vol. 150, No. 4, pp. 1341-1348.

Haubold, B. & Hudson, R.R. (2000). LIAN 3.0: detecting linkage disequilibrium in multilocus data. *Bioinformatics,* Vol. 16, No. 9, pp. 847-848.

Hudson, R.R. (1994). Analytical results concerning linkage disequilibrium in models with genetic transformation and conjugation. *Journal of Evolutionary Biology,* Vol. 7, No. 5, pp. 535-548.

Huys, G.; Kämpfer, P.; Altwegg, M.; Kersters, I.; Lamb, A.; Coopman, R.; Lüthy-Hottenstein, J.; Vancanneyt, M.; Janssen, P. & Kersters, K. (1997). *Aeromonas popoffii* sp. nov., a mesophilic bacterium isolated from drinking water production plants and reservoirs. *International Journal of Systematic Bacteriology,* Vol. 47, No. 4, pp. 1165-1171.

Huys, G.; Kämpfer, P.; Albert, M.J.; Kühn, I.; Denys, R. & Swings, J. (2002). *Aeromonas hydrophila* subsp. *dhakensis* subsp. nov., isolated from children with diarrhoea in Bangladesh, and extended description of *Aeromonas hydrophila* subsp. *hydrophila* (Chester 1901) Stanier 1943 (Approved Lists 1980). *International Journal of Systematic Bacteriology,* Vol. 52, No. 3, pp. 705-712.

Küpfer, M.; Kuhnert, P.; Korczak, B.M.; Peduzzi, R. & Demarta, A. (2006). Genetic relationships of *Aeromonas* strains inferred from 16S rRNA, *gyrB* and *rpoB* gene sequences. *International Journal of Systematic and Evolutionary Microbiology,* Vol. 56, No. 12, pp. 2743-2751.

Lan, R. & Reeves, P.R. (2001). When does a clone deserve a name? A perspective on bacterial species based on population genetics. *Trends in Microbiology,* Vol. 9, No. 9, pp. 419-424.

Levin, B.R. & Bergstrom, C.T. (2000). Bacteria are different: observations, interpretations, speculations, and opinions about the mechanisms of adaptive evolution in prokaryotes. *Proceedings of the National Academy of Sciences of the United States of America,* Vol. 97, No. 13, pp. 6981-6985.

Li, Y.; Liu, Y.; Zhou, Z.; Huang, H.; Ren, Y.; Zhang, Y.; Li, G.; Zhou, Z. & Wang, L. (2011). Complete genome sequence of *Aeromonas veronii* strain B565. *Journal of Bacteriology,* Vol. 193, No. 13, pp. 3389-3390.

Librado, P. & Rozas, J. (2009). DnaSP v5: A software for comprehensive analysis of DNA polymorphism data. *Bioinformatics,* Vol. 25, No. 11, pp. 1451-1452.

Maiden, M.C.; Bygraves, J.A.; Feil, E.; Morelli, G.; Russell, J.E.; Urwin, R.; Zhang, Q.; Zhou, J.; Zurth, K.; Caugant, D.A.; Feavers, I.M.; Achtman, M. & Spratt, B.G. (1998). Multilocus sequence typing: a portable approach to the identification of clones within populations of pathogenic microorganisms. *Proceedings of the National Academy of Sciences of the United States of America,* Vol. 95, No. 6, pp. 3140-3145.

Martin-Carnahan, A. & Joseph, S.W. (2005). Genus I. *Aeromonas* Stanier 1943, 213^{AL}, In: *Bergey's Manual of Systematic Bacteriology,* Garrity, G.M.; Brenner, D.J.; Krieg, N.R. & Staley, J.T. (eds.), Vol. 2, part B, pp. 557-578, Springer, New York.

Martínez-Murcia, A.J.; Soler, L.; Saavedra, M.J.; Chacón, M.R.; Guarro, J.; Stackebrandt, E. & Figueras, M.J. (2005). Phenotypic, genotypic, and phylogenetic discrepancies to differentiate *Aeromonas salmonicida* from *Aeromonas bestiarum*. *International Microbiology,* Vol. 8, No. 4, pp. 259-269.

Martínez-Murcia, A.J.; Saavedra, M.J.; Mota, V.R.; Maier, T.; Stackebrandt, E. & Cousin, S. (2008). *Aeromonas aquariorum* sp. nov., isolated from aquaria of ornamental fish. *International Journal of Systematic and Evolutionary Microbiology,* Vol. 58, No. 5, pp. 1169-1175.

Martínez-Murcia, A.J.; Monera, A.; Saavedra, M.J.; Oncina, R.; López-Alvarez, M.; Lara, E. & Figueras, M.J. (2011). Multilocus phylogenetic analysis of the genus *Aeromonas*. *Systematic and Applied Microbiology,* Vol. 34, No. 3, pp. 189-199.

Martino, M.E.; Fasolato, L.; Montemurro, F.; Rosteghin, M.; Manfrin, A.; Patarnello, T.; Novelli, E. & Cardazzo, B. (2011). Determination of microbial diversity of *Aeromonas* strains on the basis of multilocus sequence typing, phenotype, and presence of putative virulence genes. *Applied and Environmental Microbiology,* Vol. 77, No. 14, pp. 4986-5000.

Maynard-Smith, J. (1991). The population genetics of bacteria. *Proceedings of the Royal Society B Biological Sciences,* Vol. 245, No. 1312, pp. 37-41.

Maynard-Smith, J.; Smith, N.H.; O'Rourke, M. & Spratt, B.G. (1993). How clonal are bacteria? *Proceedings of the National Academy of Sciences of the United States of America,* Vol. 90, No. 10, pp. 4384-4388.

Maynard-Smith, J. (1995). Do bacteria have population genetics?, In: *Population Genetics of Bacteria,* Baumberg, S.; Young, J.P.W; Wellington, E.M.H. & Saunders, J.R. (eds.), pp. 1-12, Cambridge University Press, Cambridge.

McDonald, J.H. & Kreitman, M. (1991). Adaptive protein evolution at the *Adh* locus in *Drosophila*. *Nature,* Vol. 351, pp. 652-654.

Milkman, R. (1973). Electrophoretic variation in *Escherichia coli* from natural sources. *Science,* Vol. 182, No. 116, pp. 1024-1026.

Miñana-Galbis, D.; Farfán, M.; Lorén, J.G. & Fusté, M.C. (2002). Biochemical identification and numerical taxonomy of *Aeromonas* spp. isolated from environmental and clinical samples in Spain. *Journal of Applied Microbiology,* Vol. 93, No. 3, pp. 420-430.

Miñana-Galbis, D.; Farfán, M.; Fusté, M.C. & Lorén, J.G. (2004). Genetic diversity and population structure of *Aeromonas hydrophila, Aer. bestiarum, Aer. salmonicida* and

Aer. popoffii by multilocus enzyme electrophoresis (MLEE). *Environmental Microbiology,* Vol. 6, No. 3, pp. 198-208.

Miñana-Galbis, D.; Urbizu-Serrano, A.; Farfán, M.; Fusté, M.C. & Lorén, J.G. (2009). Phylogenetic analysis and identification of *Aeromonas* species based on sequencing of the *cpn60* universal target. *International Journal of Systematic and Evolutionary Microbiology,* Vol. 59, No. 8, pp. 1976-1983.

Nei, M., & Kumar, S. (2000). Genetic polymorphism and evolution, In: *Molecular Evolution and Phylogenetics,* pp. 231-264, Oxford University Press, New York.

Nhung, P.H.; Hata, H.; Ohkusu, K.; Noda, M.; Shah, M.M.; Goto, K. & Ezaki, T. (2007). Use of the novel phylogenetic marker *dnaJ* and DNA-DNA hybridization to clarify interrelationships within the genus *Aeromonas*. *International Journal of Systematic and Evolutionary Microbiology,* Vol. 57, No. 6, pp. 1232-1237.

O'Rourke, M. & Stevens, E. (1993). Genetic structure of *Neisseria gonorrhoeae* populations: a non-clonal pathogen. *Journal of General Microbiology,* Vol. 139, No. 11, pp. 2603-2611.

Orskov, F.; Whittam, T.S.; Cravioto, A. & Orskov, I. (1990). Clonal relationships among classic enteropathogenic *Escherichia coli* (EPEC) belonging to different O groups. *The Journal of Infectious Diseases,* Vol. 162, No. 1, pp. 76-81.

Pérez-Losada, M.; Brownw, E.B.; Madsen, A.; Wirth, T.; Viscidi, R.P. & Crandall, K.A. (2006). Population genetics of microbial pathogens estimated from multilocus sequence typing (MLST) data. *Infection, Genetics and Evolution,* Vol. 6, No. 2, pp. 97-112.

R Development Core Team (2010). *R: a language and environment for statistical computing,* R Foundation for Statistical Computing, Vienna, Austria, URL http://www.r-project.org/.

Reith, M.E.; Singh, R.K.; Curtis, B.; Boyd, J.M.; Bouevitch, A.; Kimball, J.; Munholland, J.; Murphy, C.; Sarty, D.; Williams, J.; Nash, J.H.E.; Johnson, S.C. & Brown, L.L. (2008). The genome of *Aeromonas salmonicida* subsp. *salmonicida* A449: insights into the evolution of a fish pathogen. *BMC Genomics,* Vol. 9, No. 427.

Roberts, M.S. & Cohan, F.M. (1993). The effect of DNA sequence divergence on sexual isolation in *Bacillus*. *Genetics,* Vol. 134, No. 2, pp. 401-408.

Robinson, A.; Falush, D. & Feil, E.J. (eds.) (2010). *Bacterial Population Genetics in Infectious Disease,* Wiley & Sons, ISBN 978-0-470-42474-2, New Yersey.

Roselló-Mora, R. & Amann, R. (2001). The species concept for prokaryotes. *FEMS Microbiology Reviews,* Vol. 25, No. 1, pp. 39-67.

Ryman, N. & Leimar, O. (2009). G_{ST} is still a useful measure of genetic differentiation - a comment on Jost's D. *Molecular Ecology.* Vol. 18, No. 10, pp. 2084-2087.

Saavedra, M.J.; Figueras, M.J. & Martínez-Murcia, A.J. (2006). Updated phylogeny of the genus *Aeromonas*. *International Journal of Systematic and Evolutionary Microbiology,* Vol. 56, No. 10, pp. 2481-2487.

Salaun, L.; Audibert, C.; Le Lay, G.; Burocoa, C.; Fauchère, J.L. & Picard, B. (1998). Panmintic structure of *Helicobacter pylori* demonstrated by the comparative study of six genetic markers. *FEMS Microbiology Letters,* Vol. 161, No. 2, pp. 231-239.

Seshadri, R.; Joseph, S.W.; Chopra, A.K.; Sha, J.; Shaw, J.; Graf, J.; Haft, D.; Wu, M.; Ren, Q.; Rosovitz, M.J.; Madupu, R.; Tallon, L.; Kim, M.; Jin, S.; Vuong, H.; Stine, O.C.; Ali, A.; Horneman, A.J. & Heidelberg, J.F. (2006). Genome sequence of *Aeromonas hydrophila* ATCC 7966: jack of all trades. *Journal of Bacteriology,* Vol. 188, No. 23, pp. 8272-8282.

Selander, R.K.; Caugant, D.A.; Ochman, H.; Musser, J.M.; Gilmour, M.N. & Whittam, T.S. (1986). Methods of multilocus enzyme electrophoresis for bacterial population genetics and systematics. *Applied and Environmental Microbiology,* Vol. 51, No. 5, pp. 873-884.

Selander, R.K.; Beltran, P.; Smith, N.H.; Helmuth, R.; Rubin, F.A.; Kopecko, D.J.; Ferris, K.; Tall, B.D.; Cravioto, A. & Musser, J.M. (1990). Evolutionary genetic relationships of clones of *Salmonella* serovars that cause human typhoid and other enteric fevers. *Infection & Immunity,* Vol. 58, No. 7, pp. 2262-2275.

Silver, A.C.; Williams, D.; Faucher, J.; Horneman, A.J.; Gogarten, J.P. & Graf, J. (2011). Complex evolutionary history of the *Aeromonas veronii* group revealed by host interaction and DNA sequence data. *PLoS ONE,* Vol. 6, No. 2, e16751.

Soler, L.; Yañez, M.A.; Chacón, M.R.; Aguilera-Arreola, M.G.; Catalán, V.; Figueras, M.J. & Martínez-Murcia, A.J. (2004). Phylogenetic analysis of the genus *Aeromonas* based on two housekeeping genes. *International Journal of Systematic and Evolutionary Microbiology,* Vol. 54, No. 5, 1511-1519.

Stackebrandt, E.; Frederiksen, W.; Garrity, G.M.; Grimont, P.A.D.; Kämpfer, P.; Maiden, M.C.J.; Nesme, X.; Rosselló-Mora, R.; Swings, J.; Trüper, H.G.; Vauterin, L.; Ward, A.C. & Whitman, W.B. (2002). Report of the *ad hoc* committee for the re-evaluation of the species definition in bacteriology. *International Journal of Systematic and Evolutionary Microbiology,* Vol. 52, No. 3, 1043-1047.

Tamura, K.; Peterson, D.; Peterson, N.; Stecher, G.; Nei, M. & Kumar, S. (2011). MEGA5: Molecular Evolutionary Genetics Analysis using Maximum Likelihood, Evolutionary Distance, and Maximum Parsimony Methods. *Molecular Biology and Evolution,* DOI: 10.1093/molbev/msr121.

Touchon, M.; Hoede, C.; Tenaillon, O.; Barbe, V.; Baeriswy, S.; Bidet, P.; Bingen, E.; Bonacorsi, S.; Bouchier, C.; Bouvet, O.; Calteau, A.; Chiapello, H.; Clermont, O.; Cruveiller, S.; Danchin, A.; Diard, M.; Dossat, C.; Karoui, M.E.; Frapy, E.; Garry, L.; Ghigo, J.M.; Gilles, A.M.; Johnson, J.; LeBouguénec, C.; Lescat, M.; Mangenot, S.; Martínez-Jéhanne, V.; Matic, I.; Nassif, X.; Oztas, S.; Petit, M.A.; Pichon, C.; Rouy, Z.; Ruf, C.S.; Schneider, D.; Tourret, J.; Vacherie, B.; Vallenet, D.; Médigue, C.; Rocha, E.P.C. & Denamur, E. (2009). Organised genome dynamics in the *Escherichia coli* species results in highly diverse adaptive paths. *PLoS Genetics,* Vol. 5, No. 1, e1000344.

Vinuesa, P.; Silva, C.; Werner, D. & Martínez-Romero, E. (2005). Population genetics and phylogenetic inference in bacterial molecular systematics: the roles of migration and recombination in *Bradyrhizobium* species cohesion and delineation. *Molecular Phylogenetics and Evolution,* Vol. 34, No. 1, pp. 29-54.

Vogel, U., Schoen, C. & Elias, J. (2010). Population genetics of *Neisseria meningitidis.* In: *Bacterial Population Genetics in Infectious Disease,* Robinson, A.; Falush, D. & Feil, E.J. (eds.), pp. 247-267, Wiley & Sons, ISBN 978-0-470-42474-2, New Yersey.

Vulic, M.; Dionisio, F.; Taddei, F. & Radman, M. (1997). Molecular keys to speciation: DNA polymorphism and the control of genetic exchange in enterobacteria. *Proceedings of the National Academy of Sciences of the United States of America,* Vol. 94, No. 18, pp. 9763-9767.

Willems, R.J. (2010). Population genetics of *Enterococcus.* In: *Bacterial Population Genetics in Infectious Disease,* Robinson, A.; Falush, D. & Feil, E.J. (eds.), pp. 195-216, Wiley & Sons, ISBN 978-0-470-42474-2, New Yersey.

Wright, S. (1940). Breeding structure of populations in relation to speciation. *American Naturalist,* Vol. 74, No. 752, pp. 232-248.

Zawadzki, P.; Roberts, M.S. & Cohan, F.M. (1995). The log-linear relationship between sexual isolation and sequence divergence in *Bacillus* transformation is robust. *Genetics,* Vol. 140, No. 3, pp. 917-932.

4

Minisatellite DNA Markers in Population Studies

Svetlana Limborska, Andrey Khrunin and Dmitry Verbenko
Institute of Molecular Genetics, Russian Academy of Sciences, Moscow Russia

1. Introduction

The discovery of an anonymous multiallelic locus in 1980 demonstrated for the first time that the human DNA contains hypervariable regions (Wyman & White, 1980). Eight alleles of a polymorphic locus that was not associated with any known gene were identified during the blot hybridization of total human genomic DNA treated with the restrictase EcoRI with a human DNA fragment (16 tbp in length) isolated from a phage genomic library. The multiallelic nature of the polymorphism at this locus did not stem from a variation in restriction sites; rather, it originated from a variable number of tandem repeats in the short core DNA sequence. Later, other similar polymorphic sites were detected near the 5′ end of the insulin gene (Bell et al., 1982), in the Harvey *ras* oncogene (Capon et al., 1983), in the ζ-globin pseudogene (Proudfoot et al., 1982), and within the β-globin cluster (Weller et al., 1984). In 1985, Jeffreys et al. published the results of their research, in which they described a fourfold repeat of 33 nucleotides in one of the introns of the human myoglobin gene (Jeffreys et al., 1985). These polymorphic regions consisted of tandem repeats of a short sequence (~11–60 bp) and were termed variable number tandem repeats (VNTRs) (Kendrew & Lawrence, 1994).

The other term for VNTR loci, minisatellites, was attributed based on the similarity of some of their properties with those of highly repetitive satellite DNA sequences. Tandem satellite DNA repeats are combined into a huge and structurally diverse group arranged into continuous clusters with monomeric units positioned in a head-to-tail configuration. The differences between minisatellite loci and satellite DNA are the greater variability in the length of the repeating unit of the latter (varying from 10 to 1000 bp) and chromosomal localization: satellite DNA is located in the regions of near-centromere heterochromatin in metaphase chromosomes and in the chromocenters of interphase nuclei, whereas minisatellite sequences are distributed evenly over most regions of all chromosomes (Miklos & John, 1979).

The classification of Jeffreys et al. discriminates between microsatellites (with an elementary link of 2–6 bp), minisatellites (up to 100 bp), midisatellites (100–400 bp), and macrosatellites (up to several thousand bp) (Jeffreys et al., 1994). Later, a great emphasis was placed on loci that were generally classified as microsatellites with elementary links of less than 10 bp (short tandem repeats, STRs) and minisatellites with links of more than 10 bp in size (VNTRs) (Schlotterer C., 1998; Gemayel et al., 2010). These two types of variable DNA were used as genetic markers in genomic and population studies.

Many minisatellites are characterized by hypervariability and a high degree of polymorphism. Their heterozygosity is 85–99%, whereas the maximum heterozygosity of biallelic loci is 50% (Bois, 2003; Gemayel et al., 2010). Minisatellite loci have been used actively in criminalistics, in the panels of highly informative markers used for the identification of individuals and ascertainment of filiation (Jurka & Gentles, 2006; Hong-Sheng et al., 2009). Data on the population frequencies of hypervariable markers were important for the determination of data reliability in such investigations (Zhivotovskii, 1996).

Minisatellite markers have also been used intensively in genetic studies, including the study of genomic diversity in human populations. However, during the last few years, because of the great technological efforts that are necessary for the typing of minisatellite markers, the main focus of population genetics research has been the investigation of short tandem repeats (STRs) and single nucleotide polymorphisms (SNPs) (Kelkar et al., 2008). Difficulties in the classification and determination of minisatellite allele variants halted the progress of the use of these DNA markers in population research. However, recently, the peculiar properties of minisatellites (i.e., new data regarding their functional significance) have rendered this class of DNA markers actual again (Babushkina & Kucher, 2011, Gemayel et al., 2010). Taking into account the high mutation rate of hypervariable minisatellites, their polymorphic nature allows not only the determination of population divergence over long periods, but also the detection of the specificity of the relatively modern (hundreds of years ago) ethnic history of populations.

2. Minisatellite loci in human DNA

The high degree of polymorphism of minisatellite sequences is evidence of the high rate of their evolution; nevertheless, most of them are rather stable. Hypermutability was demonstrated for only a few minisatellite loci (Bois, 2003). These loci are very suitable models for studying the mechanisms that lead to the variability of minisatellite sequences. Minisatellites are classified as hypermutable only when their mean mutation frequency in germ line cells is greater than 0.5%; this rate may be equal (e.g., MS1 minisatellites) or vary (e.g., CEB1 minisatellites) between male and female germ cells. According to rough estimates, less than 10 out of about 300 minisatellites typed in families were hypermutable (Amarger et al., 1998). No structural peculiarities distinguishing hypermutable minisatellites from other tandem repeats were found; the ratio of repeats with near-telomere localization to those distributed evenly over the genome was the same for minisatellites of the human genome as a whole (Vergnaud & Denoeud, 2000).

Several models have been accepted for the interpretation of the mechanisms underlying the mutational processes in minisatellite loci that result in the duplication of a repeating unit. Levinson and Gutman suggested that tandem repeat duplication occurs at random, but can be repeated many times after such an occurrence because of nonspecific mating of DNA chains resulting from replisome slippage (Levinson & Gutman, 1987). At present, this model is considered as acceptable to explain the appearance and increase in the length of microsatellites with an elementary repeat unit smaller than 10 bp (Kasai et al., 1990; Gemayel et al., 2010). The model developed by Buard and Vergnaud envisages the effect of *cis* activators on the stability of minisatellites (Buard & Vergnaud, 1994). According to this model, initiation of the recombination hotspot located outside the minisatellite structure may stimulate a perfect mosaic of intra- and interallele events. As a whole, the process appears to be an exchange that is analogous to gene conversion, with the involvement of sister chromatids. The increase of the length of minisatellites is usually polar: i.e., it consists of the addition of a new region of tandem repeats to the 3′-end region of the minisatellite. The conservativeness of the flanking regions of the minisatellite cluster is indirect evidence of the correctness of this model, whereas highly intensive reorganizations, such as intra- and interallele exchange of repeating units, occur inside the cluster (Harris, 2002).

The processes that determine the instability of minisatellites are different in somatic cells and germ line cells (Bois, 2003). The events of crossing over and gene conversion occur in the germ line, supposedly during meiosis. The somatic instability of minisatellites is determined mainly by intra-allele duplications. Figure 1 shows the events that lead to the instability of the minisatellite loci of human DNA are as follows. Moreover, the appearance of the double-stranded breaks of DNA outside the minisatellite region can lead to their migration to the minisatellite region (for a detailed review see Bois, 2003). Some models have been proposed to explain the mechanisms of this migration. The transfer of a double-stranded break results in the accumulation of mutations within the minisatellite cluster, but not in other regions of genomic DNA, which explains the hypervariability of minisatellites (Bois & Jeffreys, 1999, Bois, 2003).

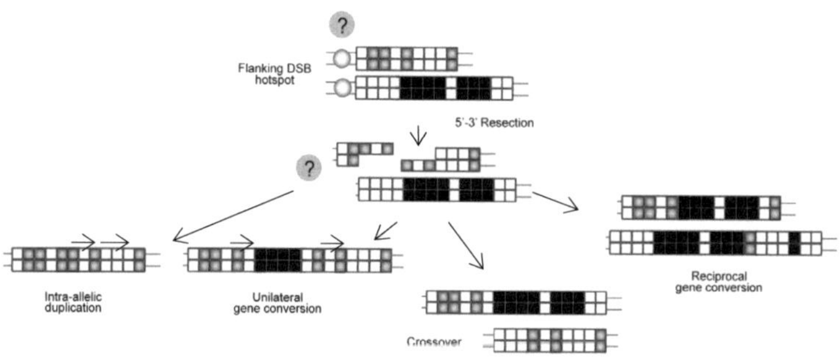

Fig. 1. Simplified model of human minisatellite instability (according to Bois, 2003). The allele destined to be mutated is shown with dark shadows, and the recipient allele is in black. An initial double strand break (DSB) outside or within minisatellite repeat can, after 5′-3′ resection, generate simple intra-alleleic duplication (no strand invasion), unilateral conversion, crossing over, or reciprocal gene conversion (strand invasion). The two steps not yet fully understood is indicated with a circled question mark. The mechanism leading to the generation of the initial DSB remain elusive. The identification of intermediates of conversion or recombination need to be characterized to dissect the various pathways. Reprinted from Genomics Vol.81, No.4, Bois, P.R. Hypermutable minisatellites, a human affair?, pp. 349-355, issn 0888-7543, Copyright 2003, with permission from Elsevier (http://www.sciencedirect.com/science/article/pii/S0888754303000211)

The availability of complete genome sequences and increased knowledge of genome biology indicate that minisatellites may occur within coding and regulatory regions, and that some minisatellites are involved in the processes of genome regulation (Gemayel et al., 2010). These sequences not only have specific biological functions, but, via their intrinsic instability, may also lead to faster rates of evolution of genes and their associated phenotypes. Variable minisatellites, as is the case for the *FLO1* gene of the benign brewer's yeast *S. cerevisiae*, lead to gradual, quantitative functional changes that may allow the rapid adaptation of the organism to changes in the environment (Verstrepen et al., 2005). Correlative observations between minisatellite allele size and gene expression patterns have been made in higher eukaryotes, including humans. One example is the minisatellite located upstream of the promoter of the human insulin gene *INS*. Shorter minisatellite alleles are linked to altered expression of *INS*, both *in vitro* and *in vivo*, and to predisposition to insulin-dependent diabetes mellitus (Bell et al., 1992; Bennett et al., 1995). Another study showed that this minisatellite affects the expression of the nearby *IGF2* gene, which encodes the insulin-like growth factor II (Paquette et al., 1999). The locus encompassing the *INS* and *IGF2* genes is termed *IDDM2*, and the minisatellite is located between the genes. The exact mechanism underlying this upregulation was not determined in the study; however, it was suggested that the tandem repeated structure of minisatellite loci might potentiate Z-DNA formation, which alters gene expression (Gemayel et al., 2010).

Several studies of human genes showed that minisatellites might interact with transcriptional factors. For example, the minisatellite located in intron 2 of the serotonin transporter gene *5-HTT* may influence its transcription levels by binding the transcription factor YB-1 (Klenova et al., 2004). The location of minisatellites involved in the regulation of gene expression and function need not be limited to promoter sequences. These loci have been found in other expression regulatory sequences, including the 5'and 3'UTRs of transcripts and introns. Many of these loci have a function in regulating gene expression, and variation in repeat units often affects their activity (Kawakami et al., 2001; Fuke et al., 2001).

Another mechanism of transcriptional regulation involves the possible interaction of miRNA with minisatellites. The unusual properties of the 27 bp minisatellite situated at exon 4 of endothelial NO synthase have been demonstrated *in vitro* using endothelial cell culture (Song et al., 2003). *eNOS* gene expression and eNOS protein concentration and enzyme activity correlate with the allele size of this VNTR. Moreover, the transcript of this VNTR is a short intronic repeat small RNA (sirRNA) that inhibits *eNOS* expression during transcription via a negative regulation mechanism (Zhang et al., 2005).

3. Hypervariable minisatellite DNA markers in human population genetics

In 1985, Jeffreys et al. published the results of their research, in which they described a minisatellite—a fourfold repeat of 33 nucleotides—in one of the introns of the human myoglobin gene (Jeffreys et al., 1985). Using this minisatellite as a probe, the authors isolated and characterized several hypervariable sequences (cores) from a human genomic library; all of these also proved to be minisatellites with 3–29 repeating units. These cores, despite their similarities to each other, exhibited some differences in their nucleotide composition and varied in length from 16 to 64 bp. They were similar in that all repeating links comprised an almost identical 15-nucleotide sequence, referred to by the authors as the core sequence, which may be described as a consensus sequence bearing certain similarities to the χ sequence of λ phage DNA (GCTGTGG). The ability of probes based on the core sequence to identify many such minisatellite loci during blot hybridization with total human DNA demonstrated the multiplicity of their localization in the genome. This property, together with the high level of polymorphism determined by the variability of the number of repeats, underscored the method of multilocus DNA fingerprinting (Jeffreys et al., 1994). Using different "policore" samples for blot hybridization, Jefferies et al. were the first to show that the hybridization pattern detected comprises many loci containing a family of minisatellites (Jeffreys et al, 1988). Blot hybridization of such sites using restricted genomic DNA revealed a picture of multiple hybridization, i.e., the presence of these loci in the genome set. The level of polymorphism of the blot hybridization patterns was extremely high, because it was determined by a combination of a large number of independent hypervariable genome loci.

Later, two independent groups of researchers, led by Ryskov in the USSR and Vassart in Belgium, discovered another family of hypervariable regions with multiple localizations in the genome, which was detected using M13 phage DNA (Ryskov et al., 1988; Dzhincharadze et al., 1987; Vassart et al., 1987). The use of two small regions that are typical of minisatellite sequences within the M13 phage DNA as a natural probe for blot hybridization with restricted DNA yielded multiple patterns of hybridization and a high level of interindividual polymorphism, which was comparable to that observed for the minisatellites described by Jeffreys et al. M13 minisatellites exhibited universal distribution in animate nature; they were found in microorganisms, plants, animals, and humans (Ryskov et al., 1988; 1990). The genomic fingerprinting technique, which analyzes many genomic polymorphic systems in the same experiment, has been used widely in forensic medicine and parentage testing (Semenova et al., 1996; Shabrova et al., 2006).

The DNA multilocus patterns determined using M13 phage hybridization were used for the first time in human population studies by Barysheva et al. (Barysheva et al.,1989, 1991a, 1991b; Semina et al., 1993). These authors determined the characteristics of M13 DNA fingerprint patterns, performed segregation analyses, and estimated the mutation frequency in M13 human minisatellite loci. The result of the cluster analysis of a genetic distance matrix confirmed data on the relationships in the group of local populations under consideration. Kalnin et al. were the first to apply multiple correspondence analysis (MCA) to the analysis of DNA fingerprinting data in human population studies (Kalnin et al., 1995). These studies demonstrated the great potential of this approach for the analysis of complex DNA multilocus blot hybridization patterns, which yield adequate results despite the inevitable errors of fragment identification that arise from the analysis of multiple autoradiographs (Shabrova et al., 2006).

However, the difficulty in analyzing DNA multilocus blot hybridization patterns, combined with the need to use the cumbersome method of blot hybridization, limited the widespread use of this approach in population genetics. Minisatellites detected later, which had unique localizations in the genome, were used widely in subsequent studies, as their detection was based on the simpler and more accessible PCR method. It eventuated that a set of singly localized (monolocus) minisatellites yielded identification patterns with an information content similar to that of the minisatellites of Jeffreys et al. or of the M13 multilocus probes. This fact favors the significant development of studies of the population characteristics of these monolocus minisatellites. The minisatellites used most frequently in population studies are those included in forensic identification panels, the most popular of which are the 3'APOB and D1S80 minisatellites; the properties of these minisatellites will be addressed in detail.

4. The 3′APOB minisatellite polymorphism in human population research

One of the VNTR loci maps to chromosome 2 and is located 75 bp from the second polyadenylation signal at the 3′ end of the *APOB* gene (Huang &Breslow, 1987). The APOB protein is one of the major low-density lipoproteins and plays a central role in the metabolism of serum cholesterol. The 3′*APOB* hypervariable region consists of a tandem-repeat sequence that is rich in A and T. Two basic types of 15-nucleotide-long core repeats have been identified (Buresi et al., 1996). The tandem repeating unit of the 3′*APOB* minisatellite consists of two tandem sequences of 14 and 16 bp; thus, neighboring allelic variants differ from each other by 30 bp, or by 2 repeats. Allelic variants differ in the number of repeats and contain 25 to 55 repeat units (Ludwig et al., 1989). The literature describes several systems of alleles for the 3′*APOB* locus. Since the establishment of one such system by Ludwig, allelic variants are denoted as 30, 32, 34, etc., according to the number of repeated units. According to the system of Boerwinkle (Boerwinkle et al., 1989), which counts one structure-segment sequence before the minisatellite cluster, the same allelic variants are designated as 31, 33, 35, etc., respectively. Thus, the allelic variant with number 36 of Ludwig's system corresponds to variant 37 of Boerwinkle's system. In addition to the two types of core segment structure, the 3′*APOB* alleles of a number of core segments have sequence microvariations (a pure AT sequence is interrupted by a C or a G), usually concentrated at the 3′ end of the minisatellite (Chen et al., 1999; Marz et al., 1993; Buresi et al., 1996). In the human population samples analyzed by Buresi et al., a haplotype analysis of such substitutions revealed the presence of five allelic sequences. The authors found the ancestral state of the 3′*APOB* minisatellite allelic sequence via comparison with another allele sequence variant discovered in primates and showed that different types of allele sequences in humans appeared during 3′*APOB* minisatellite evolution due to three possible conversions at the minisatellite locus (Buresi et al., 1996).

The 3′APOB polymorphism has been used widely in investigations of the history and diversity of humans, both worldwide and in individual population groups (Buresi et al., 1996; Destro-Bisol et al., 2000; Renges et al., 2002; Kravchenko et al., 1996; Poltl et al., 1996; Zago et al., 1996; Verbenko et al., 2005). It has been considered as a suitable locus for a pilot study of the relationships between the shape of allele-size distributions of minisatellites and the microevolutionary processes leading to their present-day distribution (Destro-Bisol et al., 2000). The allele-size frequencies can be used to calculate interpopulation genetic distances. Higher differences in the level of polymorphism have been found in populations with different origins and ethnicities (Buresi et al., 1996; Destro-Bisol et al., 2000; Renges et al., 2002; Kravchenko et al., 1996; Poltl et al., 1996).

The use of the 3′*APOB* minisatellite as a marker in the study of evolutionary models was launched in 1992 (Renges et al., 2002). Subsequently, scientists from many countries studied the 3′*APOB* minisatellite polymorphism in a large number of human populations. Although the allele frequencies vary considerably among different populations, the similarities in their distribution shapes should be noted. Generally, two allelic variants (34 and 36 repeats) are detected most often (their total frequency is 57–77%), one or two allelic variants are less frequent (usually a variant containing 32, 46, or 48 repetitions, with frequencies up to 12%), whereas other alleles occur with a frequency of less than 5% (Boerwinkle et al, 1989a; Ludwig et al., 1989; Deka et al., 1992; Friedl et al., 1990; Renges et al., 1992; Lahermo et al.,

1996; Spitsyn et al., 2000; Destro-Bisol et al., 2000; Khusnutdinova et al., 1999; Khusnutdinova and et al. 2003; Akhmetov et al, 2006; Bermisheva et al., 2007). As an example, we considered the population characteristics of the 3'*APOB* polymorphism in Eastern European populations.

Eastern Europe is inhabited by a great number of ethnic groups that differ significantly in their characteristics (Kuzeev, 1985; Bunak, 1965). East Slavs are the main population group in Eastern Europe. The formation of East Slavic peoples (Russians, Ukrainians, and Belarusians) is supposed to have occurred because of the long-term migration and expansion of ancestral Slav tribes from Central Europe to the territory of the Russian Plain, which was settled by pre-Finno-Ugric tribes, since the Late Paleolithic (Sedov, 1979; Alekseeva, 1973). Ethnic groups of the southern region and surrounding Ural Mountains, which neighbor the East Slavic peoples, have an even more luxuriant history resulting in the formation of the Turkic language groups of Tatars and Bashkirs, the peoples of the North Caucasus, and Mongoloid populations such as the Kalmyks.

The Eastern Slavonic linguistic group (Indo-European linguistic family) was represented by samples from Russian populations from the European (northwestern) part of Russia (Oschevensk, Belaia Sluda, Kholmogory, Mezen, Kursk, Novgorod, Cossacks, Sychevka, Kostroma, and Smolensk), and six Byelorussian populations (Grodno, Pinsk, Mjadel, Bobruisk, Nesvij, and Khoiniki) from different regions of the Republic of Belarus (for a detailed description of the Byelorussians, see Popova *et al.* (Popova et al., 2001). The Belaia Sluda group is an isolated Russian population living at the border of the Arkhangelsk region of northern Russia with the Republic of Komi. The Oschevensk group is an isolated Russian population living in the Kargopol district of the Arkhangelsk region. From ethnohistorical and anthropological points of view, these Russian groups might carry an admixture of ancient Vepsian (Ageeva, 2000) or Saami lineages (Sedov, 1979; Alekseeva, 1973). The Kholmogory are based in a town near the city of Arkhangelsk, representing Russian north-coast dwellers, and the Mezen group is from the same lineage, which is derived from Russians who migrated from Novgorod to the northeast, starting in the 16th century. The Novgorod group is from the northwestern European part of Russia. The Kursk group is a southwestern Russian population. The Cossacks are a southern Russian population from the Krasnodar region (settled at the Kuban River). The Smolensk group is from the town of Ugra, with a complex history of population movements (southwestern part of Eastern Europe), and the Sychevka group is also from the Smolensk district of Russia (from the central part of the Russian Plain, which borders the Tver district).

Populations from the western Ural region were represented by Finno-Ugric speakers—the Komi-Permyats from the Perm district of Russia, the Komi-Ziryans (Izhemski and Priluszki Komi subpopulations), the Udmurts, and the Meadow Maris—and by Turkic speakers (Altaic linguistic family): the Bashkirs, from the Beloretsky region of the Republic of Bashkiria, and the Tatars, from the town of Almetyevsk (for a detailed description of these groups see Bermisheva *et al.*, 2003). The Komi (Komi-Zyryans) are one of the most numerous peoples of the Finno-Ugrian group: they occupy the northeasternmost location among European ethnic groups, which adjacent to the Nentsy. They inhabit the territory of the basins and the tributaries of the Vichegda, Mezen and Pechora rivers. The contemporary Komi people consist of some distinct ethnographic groups, which formed during the 8th to the 19th centuries. Two geographically different ethnographic groups were studied in this work. One of them, the Izhemski Komi, takes a particular place among the Komi groups. They stand out because of a number of peculiarities of their language and traditional economy. The latter has long been based on the commodity of reindeer breeding. Moreover, the Izhemski Komi exhibit some anthropological traits that differentiate them from other Komi groups. Unlike the Izhemski Komi, the Priluzski Komi have traditionally occupied themselves with farming and cattle breeding. In addition, the Priluzski Komi belong to ethnic groups that, historically, formed before the Izhemski Komi people. Two ethnic groups originate from the Altaic linguistic family, but do not inhabit the Ural region: these are the Kalmyk and Yakut populations. Kalmyks inhabit the steppe region located to the northwest of the Caspian Sea. This ethnic group settled in their current region of inhabitance during a migration from the Dzungaria region of Central Asia in the 16th century (northwestern China). The Yakut population lives in East Siberia and belongs to the Turkic linguistic group (Altaic linguistic family). In classical anthropology, they are classified as the Central Asian type (Cavalli-Sforza et al., 1994). In this study, samples from the Elista region of Kalmykia and from a central group of Yakut people were examined.

The blood samples used in this study were obtained by venipuncture into EDTA-coated Vacutainer tubes after obtaining informed consent from each individual. To fulfill the selection criteria, all individuals had to belong to the native ethnic group of the region studied (descended from at least three generations living in the region), be unrelated to each other, and be healthy. DNA isolation and purification, PCR analysis, gel electrophoresis, and multidimensional statistical analyses were performed as described in Verbenko et al (Verbenko et al., 2003a, 2006). Calculations of population characteristics, pairwise genetic distances, and molecular variances were performed using POPGENE version 1.32 (Yeh et al., 1999) and GDA (Weir, 1996, Lewis & Zaykin, 2001) software. Fisher's exact testing of contingency tables was performed using RxC software (Miller, 1997). The phylogenetic interrelation in the populations of Eastern Europe was studied based on data on the variability of these minisatellite loci, and genetic distances were calculated according to Nei (Nei, 1972). The matrix obtained was used for analysis using the method of multidimensional scaling, which visualizes interrelations between the populations and facilitates the significant interpretation of results, especially regarding the multimodal distribution of the frequencies of allele variants.

The data obtained revealed the presence of 31 allelic variants of the 3'*APOB* minisatellite, ranging in size from 24 to 54 repetitions with varying frequency in the population. Nine (in a population of Meadow Mari) to 17 (in a population of Bobruisk Belarusians) different alleles were found in different populations. A wide range of variability in 3'*APOB* minisatellite alleles indicates a high level of polymorphism in the populations under study. In the Eastern European populations studied here, the most frequent allelic variants of the 3'*APOB* minisatellite had 34 and 36 repeats. The allele with 36 repeats is dominant in European populations of Eastern Slavs (Russian, Belarusian, and Ukrainian), whereas the allele with 34 repeats is most frequent in the Asian populations (Kalmyk and Yakut). This is consistent with the results of the majority of the works addressing the variability of this marker in populations worldwide. Major allelic variants represent the largest contribution to the peculiarity of allele frequency differences in the populations; however, a wide range of information stems from minor allelic variants containing 30, 32, 38, 40, or 42 repeats, which contribute to the identity of particular groups and specific populations.Modality is a peculiarity of the distribution of allele frequencies at the 3'*APOB* minisatellite locus, which can be treated as the main human-group diagnostic feature. The histogram (Figure 2) displays the allele frequency distributions of the 3'*APOB* minisatellite in populations of Russians, Yakuts, and Africans (Cameroon) (Destro- Bisol et al., 2000). The pronounced differences in the distribution of the major alleles containing 34 and 36 repeats can be observed. In contrast to those observed for European and Asian populations, the profile of the allele frequency distribution in populations of sub-Saharan African origin is unimodal (Deka et al., 1992; Renges et al., 1992; Destro-Bisol et al., 2000).

The allele spectrum of the 3'*APOB* minisatellite in Eastern European populations (Russians, Belarusians, Ukrainians, Adygeis, Circassians, and Abkhazians) is bimodal, with peaks at alleles 34–36 and 48. In contrast, the Asian populations of Kalmyk and Yakut and the population of the Volga–Ural region do not exhibit the second peak; the frequency distribution of the allelic variants observed in these populations is unimodal.

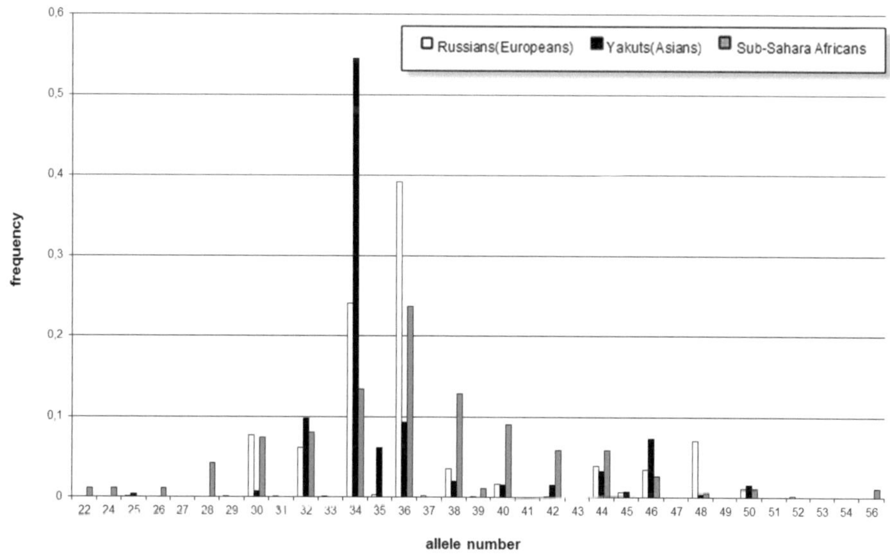

Fig. 2. 3'-end APOB minisatellite allele frequency distributions in populations of three main human groups.

A comparative analysis of the data obtained with European and Asian population data from literature revealed the similarity between the Eastern Slavs and the European populations of western and central Europe, and the Yakut and Kalmyk - with Asian populations (Chinese and Japanese) (Verbenko et al., 2003a). The analysis of the data using multidimensional scaling showed two clusters: Asian and European, which has a compact core. At the heart of the European population cluster were Germans, French, Swedish, Russians, Ukrainians, and Belarusians. The proximity of the East Slavic populations to the main Western Europeans supports the view of archaeologists and anthropologists regarding a Central European origin for the Eastern Slavs. According to this type of research, the ancestral home of the Slavs was settled between the Oder and the Vistula (Sedov, 1979 as cited in Verbenko et al., 2003a).

The Figure 3 shows the results of multidimensional scaling of Nei's pairwise genetic distances calculated for Eastern European populations. The resulting graph can be interpreted as both first and second dimensions, and considering the axes together. Based on the first dimension, it should be noted that a core group of populations inhabiting Eastern Europe is concentrated at the origin of the coordinates, whereas the populations with Asian origin of Kalmyk and Yakut are visibly removed from it. A common alliance of Eastern Slavs (Russian, Ukrainian, and Byelorussian populations), Northern Caucasians (Adygeys—including Adygei-Shapsugs of the Black Sea coast—Abkhasians, and Circassian populations), and populations living close to the Ural Mountains region (Komis, Bashkirs, and Mari) may be distinguished further taking into account the second dimension.

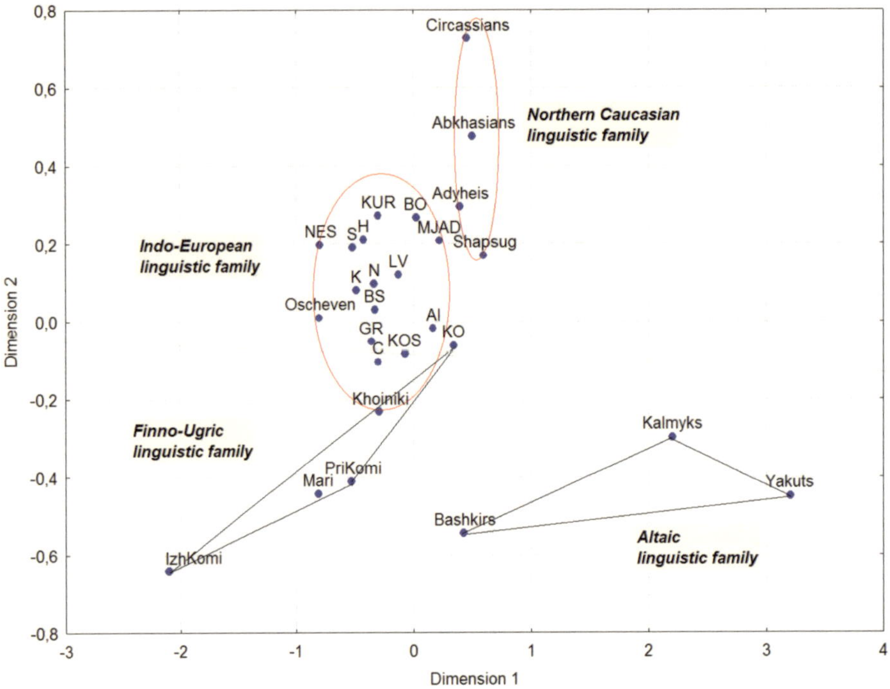

Fig. 3. Multidimensional scaling plot (two dimensions) of Nei's genetic distances among 26 populations of Eastern Europe and one population from Siberia based on 3'APOB minisatellite variability. Linguistic affiliations of populations are designated with geometrical figures. Abbreviations are: Russians: Cossacks (C), Belaya Sluda (BS), Kholmogory (H), Kostroma (KOS), Novgorod (N), Oschevensk (Osheven), Smolensk (S), Kursk (KUR); Belarussians: Grodno (GR), Khoiniki, Nesvij (NES), Mjadel' (MJAD), Bobruisk (BO); Ukrainians: Kiev (K), Lviv (LV), Alchevsk (AL); Other ethnic groups: Circassians, Abkhazians, Adygeis, Shapsugs (North Caucasus geographic region); Bashkirs (Beloretsky region), Komi-Permyats (KO), Izhemski Komi (IzKomi), Priluzski Komi (PriKomi), Maris (Ural geographic region), Kalmyks, Yakuts.

If the linguistic classification of populations is taken into account, Eastern Slavonic, Northern Caucasian, Altaic, and Finno-Ugric clusters can be assigned. Within the main cluster of Eastern Slavs, discrete Russian, Ukrainian (Kravchenko et al., 1996), and Belarusian populations can be differentiated easily. Despite their wide geographical distribution, the Eastern Slavonic populations (Russians, Ukrainians, and Byelorussians) have a common historical lineage and are also closely associated according to their 3'*APOB* polymorphisms. For example, although Kuban Cossacks (an ethnic community of Russians from the Krasnodar region) inhabit part of the Northern Caucasus, they are closer to the Eastern Slavonic populations than to other populations of their locality. The closest relationships among the Eastern Slavonic linguistic group are between the Russian and Ukrainian populations. The greatest diversity is found for the Byelorussian populations, which are distributed around other Eastern Slavonic populations on the plot. This diversity was possibly caused by long-term gene flow during numerous migrations through the Belarus region.

The cluster of the Finno-Ugric linguistic family and the Northern Caucasian linguistic family are close to the Eastern Slavonic linguistic group cluster. The Bashkirs belong to the Altaic language family, although their localization in the graph is close to the populations of the Finno-Ugric language family. However, there is some level of proximity of the Bashkir population to other peoples of the Altaic language family (the Kalmyk and Yakut). The position of Komi-Permyats, in this case in the immediate vicinity of the Eastern Slavonic populations, alienates them from the populations living close to the Ural Mountains region and may be due to the peculiarities of the ethnic history of the Komi-Permyats (Bunak, 1965; Kuzeev, 1985). We know that this ethnic group was separated from the Komi people only a few centuries ago, and is characterized recently by very close contact with Eastern Slavonic populations, which apparently left an imprint on the formation of the gene pool of the Komi-Permyats. The special arrangement of the Izhemski Komi, which alienates them from other groups, may also be due to the peculiarities of the ethnic history of this group (Khrunin et al., 2007).We found similar 3'*APOB* diversity among Eastern Slavonic and Northern Caucasus ethnic groups. However, there were significant differences for the Kalmyk and Yakut populations of Asian origin, as well as for Uralic Komis, Mari, and Bashkirs. The differences observed are similar to those obtained based on other DNA polymorphisms (Belyaeva et al., 1999, 2003; Bermisheva et al., 2001; Khar'kov et al., 2004; Kravchenko et al., 2002; Malyarchuk et al., 2001, 2002; Mirabal et al., 2009; Orekhov et al., 1999; Popova et al., 1999, 2001; Shabrova et al., 2004) and are in good agreement with ethnohistorical (Ageeva, 2000) and anthropological data (Alexeeva, 1973, Sedov, 1979). These observations underscore the significance of the 3'*APOB* minisatellite locus for population genetics research.

Thus, the 3'*APOB* minisatellite locus exhibits decreased genetic heterogeneity among 16 broadly distributed Eastern Slavonic populations, in contrast with its significant heterogeneity among Northern Caucasian populations and among Altaic and Finno-Ugric-speaking populations. This peculiarity may reflect the integrity of the Eastern Slavonic gene pool and suggests negligible influences from neighboring ethnic groups during the process of origin and differentiation of Eastern Slavs at the 3'*APOB* genome site. At the same time, the genotype frequency distribution revealed significant differences between Eastern Slavonic groups—both among the ethnic groups and between closely related populations belonging to one ethnic group that reveals high-differentiation properties of this marker.

5. D1S80 minisatellite polymorphism in human population research

The hypervariable minisatellite locus D1S80 (pMCT118) is the second most frequently used marker in population studies; it is located in the short arm of chromosome 1 and is a tandemly organized repeating region with an elementary link of 16 bp (Nakamura et al, 1988).

D1S80 is located at a distance of 16.5 kb from the start of the gene that encodes the η2 subunit of phospholipase, which plays an important role in the calcium metabolism of cerebral neurons, but no imbalance due to coupling between D1S80 region and the sequence of this gene has been found (Jeffreys et al, 1985; Sajantila et al., 1992; Tanaka, 2005). The allele variants of D1S80 vary in length because of variable repetition of the elementary link (15 to 41 or more repeats). According to the notation of alleles by Nakamura et al. (Nakamura et al, 1988), different alleles are designated in compliance with the number of repeats. The spectrum and frequencies of D1S80 alleles have been described fairly comprehensively, as this locus has been used intensively in criminalistics and forensic medical examinations (Kasai et al., 1990). Subsequently, Budowle et al. suggested the possibility of using D1S80 to differentiate populations (Budowle et al., 1991, 1995). The first investigation of the variability of this locus on a global scale, namely, in 43 populations from different regions of the world, was published by Duncan et al. in 1996 (Duncan et al., 1996-97). Clear distinctions were noted between populations of different main human groups and high similarity was shown among populations of the same main human group.

The subsequent report of a global analysis of D1S80 variability, performed by Mastana and Papiha (Mastana & Papiha, 2001), described the study of the marker in 84 world populations. The authors presented the spectra of D1S80 allele frequencies and, using the method of factor correspondence analysis, revealed clear-cut distinctions between European, Asian, Afro-American, American Indian, and Indian ethnic groups. Subsequently, the D1S80 polymorphism was analyzed in 33 world populations with a focus on the variability of the marker in sub-Saharan African populations (aboriginals of Africa) and a population of Arabian origin (the population of Egypt) (Herrera et al., 2004). As the differentiation of ethnic groups based on D1S80 data provided a very good description of the peculiarities of the groups, which were demonstrated previously via the analysis of biochemical markers, and conforms with the geographical locations of the populations with the peculiarities of their origin, the authors drew a conclusion allowing the applicability of only one marker, D1S80, to the study of the phylogenetic interrelationships of populations (Herrera et al., 2004).

A multimodal distribution is the distinctive feature of the spectrum of D1S80 allele frequencies. Some D1S80 alleles occur quite frequently, e.g., the total frequency of allele variants with 18 and 24 repeats is as high as 70% (Das & Mastana, 2003, Herrera et al., 2004, Walsh & Eckhoff , 2007). The first major allele, which contains 18 repeat units, occurs in 5.5–9% of sub-Saharan African populations, in 15–21% of Asian populations, and in 13–35% of European populations. The second major allele (24 repeats) has a frequency of 26–45% in Europeans, 6–29% in sub-Saharan Africans, and 17–24% in Asians(Das & Mastana, 2003; Duncan et al., 1996-97; Budowle et al., 1991, 1995; Herrera et al., 2004; Sajantila et al., 1992).

Some of the allele variants may either have a very high or very low frequency in particular populations, or even in the main human groups. Thus, in comparison with other main human groups, sub-Saharan Africans are characterized by very high frequencies of alleles 17 (up to 10%), 21 (up to 16%), 22 (up to 12%), 28 (up to 20%), and 34 (up to 31%), and a low frequency of allele 18. Moreover, the diversity of the aboriginal groups of Africa is so high that each population has its own typical profile of distribution with different numbers of repeats and positions of modes (modal values). This picture is also typical for the aboriginals of northern Australia.

We studied the polymorphism of the D1S80 minisatellite in 32 populations from the Eastern European region (Verbenko et al., 2003b, 2004, 2006, 2007; Khrunin et al., 2007; Limborska et al., 2011a). The study revealed the presence of 27 allele variants of the D1S80 minisatellite, with sizes ranging from 15 to more than 41 repeats and with varying frequencies in these populations. Various populations of Eastern Europe have 11 (in Ukrainians from Lviv (Kravchenko et al., 2001) and Byelorussians from Nesvij) to 20 (in Kalmyks) different allele variants. The broad spectrum of variability observed for the alleles of the D1S80 minisatellite provides evidence of the high level of polymorphism present in the populations under study. Though the allele frequencies vary significantly in different populations, their common features can be traced in their distribution. As a rule, three alleles (with 18, 24, and 31 repeats) occur at maximal frequency (the total frequency of their occurrence is 50–75%), one or two alleles occur more rarely (usually, these are variants containing 22, 25, 28, and 30 repeats, with frequencies of up to 11%), whereas other alleles usually occur with a frequency of less than 5%. Allele 24 is predominant in the European populations of Eastern Slavs (Russians, Belarusians, and Ukrainians) and allele 18 predominates in the populations of Kalmyks and Yakuts, which have an Asian origin. The populations of the Volga–Ural region (Tatars, Udmurts, Bashkirs, Maris, and Komis) and the populations of the Adygei–Abkhazia group (Adygeis, Abkhazians, and Circassians) have approximately the same frequencies of alleles 18 and 24. The frequency of allele 31 is low in European populations, intermediate in Asians, and maximal (up to 17%) in some populations of the Volga–Ural region.

The distribution of D1S80 allele frequencies in the populations studied is multimodal (see examples in Figure 4). The spectrum of alleles in European (Russian), Asian (Yakut), and Uralic (Udmurt) populations has common maxima for alleles 18 and 24. The ratio of the frequencies of alleles 18 and 24 is unequal among populations of the main human groups; the phenomenon of inversion of the frequency of the major alleles 18 and 24 is particularly noticeable between Asian and European populations. The comparison of D1S80 allele frequency distributions between the populations studied and worldwide populations revealed a similarity between Central European populations and Eastern Slavs, and between Yakut and Kalmyk populations and other Asian populations of China and Japan (Verbenko et al., 2006).

The capacity of minisatellite D1S80 to differentiate Eastern European populations was studied using multidimensional scaling of Nei's genetic distance matrix based on D1S80 allele distributions (Fig. 5, mathematical space). The main group including the Eastern Slav and Adygei–Abkhazian populations is concentrated in the cluster to the right of the origin of coordinates; the genetic relationship of these two groups can be interpreted easily based on their common European origin. Thus, European populations form one of the main clusters on the multidimensional scaling plot. Populations with an Asian origin (Kalmyks and Yakuts) are characterized by significant remoteness from Europeans. Populations of the Ural geographic region (Udmurts, Maris, Komis, Bashkirs, and Tatars) are located to the right of the origin of coordinates, in an intermediate position between the European and Asian populations. The second dimension provides the distinct differentiation between the populations that live close to the region of the Ural Mountains and the populations with an Asian origin.

The grouping of populations according to linguistic classification is indicated in the Figure 5. The populations of the Eastern Slavonic linguistic family (Russians, Ukrainians, and

Belarusians) form a single cluster, which also includes the populations of the Northern Caucasian linguistic family, as a subcluster. Russian populations from the Arkhangelsk region (Oschevensk and Belaya Sluda settlements), which are located within the cluster of the Finno-Ugric linguistic group, are the exception. The peculiar positions of these populations may be a reflection of peculiarities in their ethnic history regarding the variability of the D1S80 minisatellite; they were formed in the course of the development of northern lands by Russians under the active assimilation of native Finno-Ugric peoples, starting from the second millennium AD. This fact seems to have left a mark on the formation of their gene pool. A comparison of these findings with the results obtained in the study of mitochondrial DNA and Y chromosome markers revealed the corresponding peculiarities of these populations. Thus, a detailed analysis of the combination of nine polymorphic restriction sites with mutations of the first hypervariable segment of the mitochondrial DNA of the Russian population of Oschevensk in the Arkhangelsk region revealed a high frequency of the U5b1 mitotype, which is typical of the Finno-Ugric population of Lapps (Belyaeva et al, 2003; Balanovsky et al, 2008; Limborska et al., 2011b). An analysis of the haplotypes of Y chromosome microsatellite markers in the populations of Eastern Slavs demonstrated the kinship between these populations; only the population of Oschevensk in the Arkhangelsk region was characterized by a special set of haplotypes. Comparison of these findings with the variability of Y chromosome haplotypes in European populations revealed the kinship between the Arkhangelsk population from Oschevensk and not only Slavic, but also Finno-Ugric populations (Khrunin et al., 2005). The analysis of the data of mitochondrial DNA and Y chromosome polymorphisms, taking into consideration the peculiarities of ethnic history, leads to the conclusion that the gene pools of some Russian populations from the Arkhangelsk region contain an ancestral Finno-Ugric component.

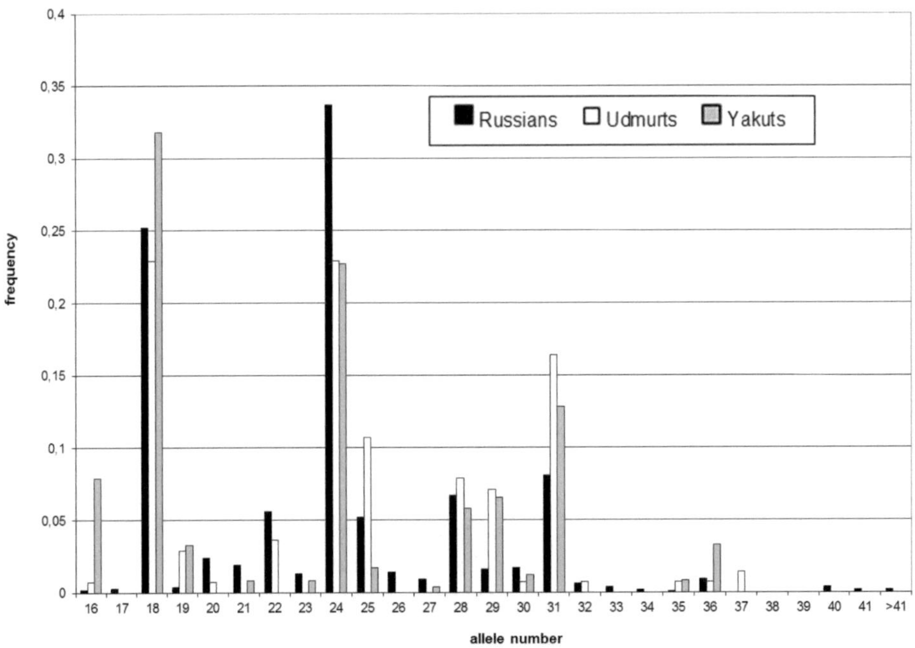

Fig. 4. D1S80 minisatellite allele frequency distributions in populations from Russia.

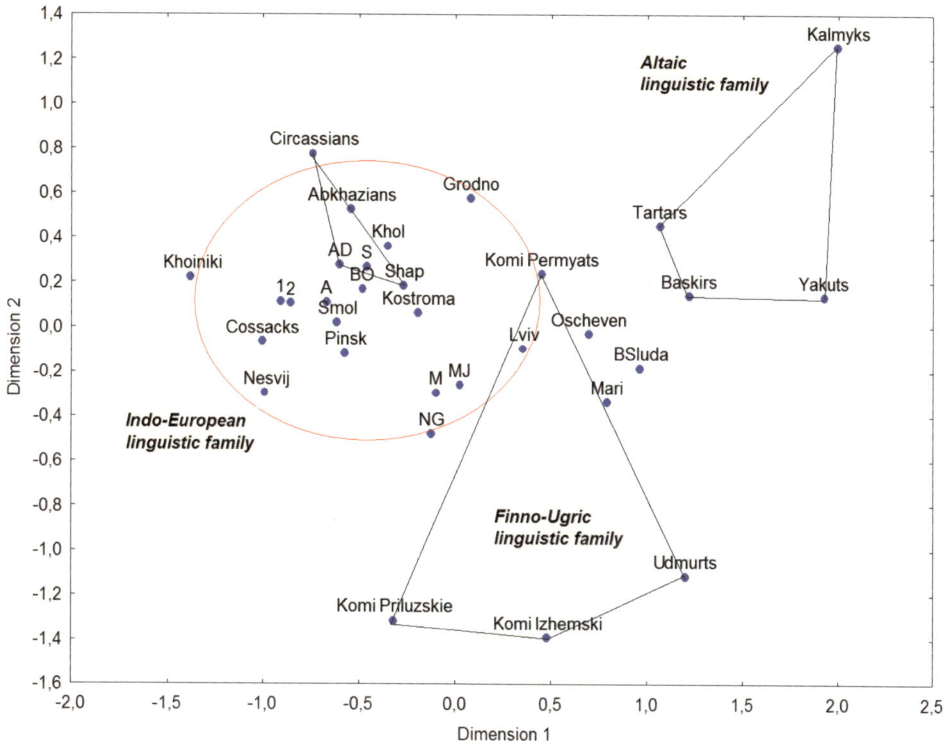

Fig. 5. Multidimensional scaling plot (two dimensions) of Nei's genetic distances among 31 populations of Eastern Europe and one population from Siberia. Linguistic affiliations of populations are designated with geometrical figures. The triangle includes the populations of North Caucasus linguistic family (except for Russians). Abbreviations are: European origin populations: Circassians, Abkhazians, Adygeis (AD), Shapsugs (Shap) (North Caucasus geographic region); Russians: Cossacks, Belaya Sluda (BSluda), Kholmogory (Khol), Kostroma, Novgorod (NG), Oschevensk (Osheven), Mezen (M), Smolensk (Ugra district) (Smol), Smolensk (Sychevka district) (S), Kursk (1); Belarussians: Grodno, Khoiniki, Nesvij, Mjadel' (MJ), Bobruisk (BO), Pinsk; Ukrainians: Kiev (2), Lviv, Alchevsk (A); Circassians, Abkhazians, Adygeis (AD), Shapsugs (Shap) (North Caucasus geographic region); Other ethnic groups: Bashkirs, Tartars, Komi-Permyats, Izhemski Komi, Priluzski Komi, Udmurts, Maris (Ural geographic region), Kalmyks, Yakuts.

Based on the aforementioned data, we can conclude that there is a spectrum of distribution of allele frequencies of specific alleles of D1S80 for the main human groups and for individual populations. It should be noted that the nature of the variability of this minisatellite differs from that of the 3'*APOB* minisatellite locus; however, both represent markers that can be used to differentiate clearly the major human groups and identify the peculiarities of individual populations. A good example is the case of the Russian populations of European origin that live in the Arkhangelsk district: the Oschevensk and the Belaia Sluda. These two populations from the same ethnic group can be readily distinguished from other Russian populations using multidimensional scaling of the D1S80 minisatellite variability genetic distance matrix, whereas the 3'*APOB* minisatellite, which is located in a different chromosome, does not differentiate these populations among other Russians. One can propose that the characteristics of 3'*APOB* and D1S80 reflect different aspects of the history of population evolution.

Thus, the minisatellite DNA markers 3'*APOB* and D1S80 are sensitive and informative markers that can be applied to the study of the genetic structure of populations and population differences, and can be used to determine the genetic affinities among populations and to reconstruct their evolutionary relationships. The minisatellites D1S80 and 3'*APOB* have been used extensively in population studies worldwide. Analysis of these loci in the population of Russia is an important part of population studies, both in terms of describing the variability of the gene pool, and as an annex to the global analysis of the origin and differentiation of human populations.

6. Allele spectrum shape subdivision using the SNP–VNTR haplotype at D1S80

To explore the evolutionary scenario underlying the complex allele distribution shape of D1S80 in different populations, we used an innovative technique of simultaneous determination of SNPs and minisatellites (Limborska et al., 2011a). Using fluorescently labeled primers and fragment analysis via capillary electrophoresis, we identified a hypervariable combination of the minisatellite polymorphism at the D1S80 locus and a SNP (G>T, rs16824398) adjacent to (74 bp) the minisatellite. The approach applied allows the determination of autosomal haplotypes representing the combinations of VNTR alleles with certain repeat numbers and alleles of the flanking SNP (Figure 6). A comparison of the SNPrs1682498-D1S80 haplotype frequencies was performed in populations of European (Russians), Asian (Yakuts), and African origin (from the sub-Saharan region; student volunteers from the Peoples' Friendship University of Russia, Moscow).

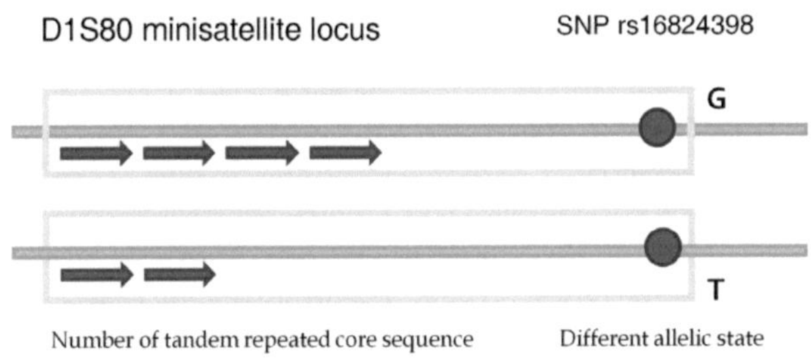

Fig. 6. Schematic of SNP-VNTR system (hypervariable minisatellite polymorphism combination of locus D1S80 and a single-nucleotide polymorphism) depicting double heterozygote autosomal haplotype for a diploid organism. In this example, one homolog has a G allele at the SNP and minisatellite locus of four (as e.g.) repeat units. The other homolog has a T allele at the SNP and minisatellite locus of two (as e.g.) repeat units.

The distributions of D1S80 allele frequencies in the populations studied are shown in Figures 7-9. Twenty-two alleles containing 16–41 repeats were detected among the 820 chromosomes typed. The allele spectra of all populations were multimodal, with the main peaks at alleles 18 and 24 in the Russian and Yakut samples. The frequency of allele 24 was high in the two Russian populations and the frequency of allele 18 was highest among the

Yakuts. The African allele spectrum was expanded and had peaks at alleles 18 and 24, albeit at lower frequency; the other major alleles were alleles 21 and 28.

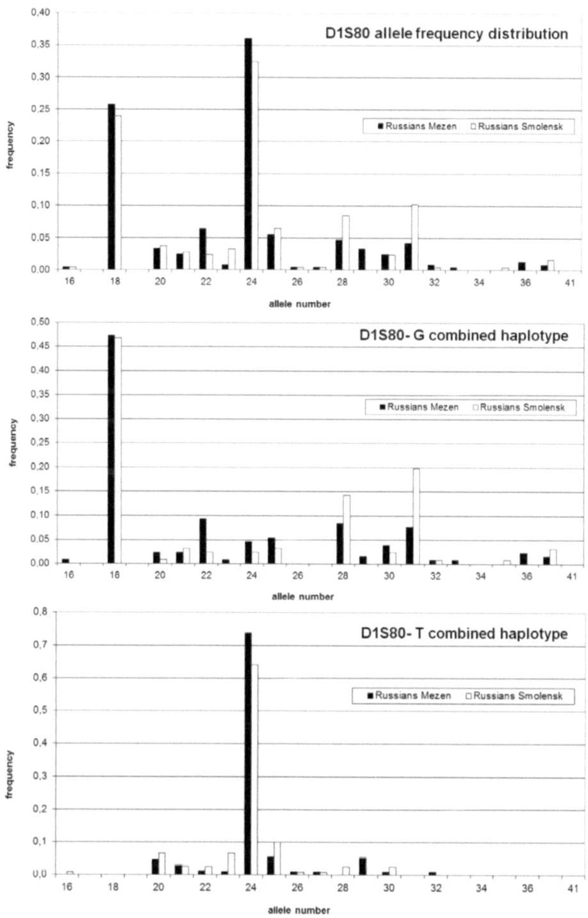

Fig. 7. D1S80 minisatellite allele frequency distributions in two geographically Russian populations (Europeans).

An analysis of the amplified SNPrs1682498-D1S80 allelic pairs revealed the chromosome-related specificity of D1S80 allele spectra. A likelihood-ratio test was used to assess the significance of the LD between each D1S80 allele and SNP alleles. One of the most frequent variants, allele 24, was significantly associated with the T allele in non-African samples (D′ = 0.75–0.93; $P < 1 \times 10^{-4}$). This combination was 10 times more frequent than the combination including the G allele. No significant association between allele 24 and the SNP background was observed in the African group, in which both combinations occurred almost equally (20.5% and 15.1%, respectively; D′ = 0.11; $P = 0.465$). In Africans, the T allele was associated most strongly with allele 21. This combination also occurred 10 times more frequently than the combination including the G allele. Another frequent D1S80 allele containing 18 repeats was in complete LD (D′ = 1.00) with the G allele and was not detected on the T background in any of the populations. However, it occurred about three times more frequently in non-

African populations (40.4–47.3%) than in African samples. The other common D1S80 alleles (28 and 31) and population-specific alleles (e.g., 16 in Yakuts and 33 in Africans) were also associated mainly with the G allele. One exception was allele 31 among the Yakuts, which had no specific linkage with any of the SNP alleles (G, 12.3%; T, 10.9%; D′ = 0.09; $P = 0.785$).

Generally, the African samples showed greater genetic diversity for each SNP allele background than did the samples from the other populations. Lower values of allele diversity were estimated on the T background in each population. This could be explained by the observation that most D1S80 alleles were less frequent on the T background, and that the absolute number of alleles was also lower compared with that observed for the G background (including the absence of alleles with more than 32 repeats on the T background). A comparison of the SNP-linked D1S80 allele distributions between pairs of populations revealed a high degree of similarity ($P > 0.01$) among the allele spectra on the T background in non-African samples. In the case of the G-background-related distributions, a similarity was evident only among Russian samples.

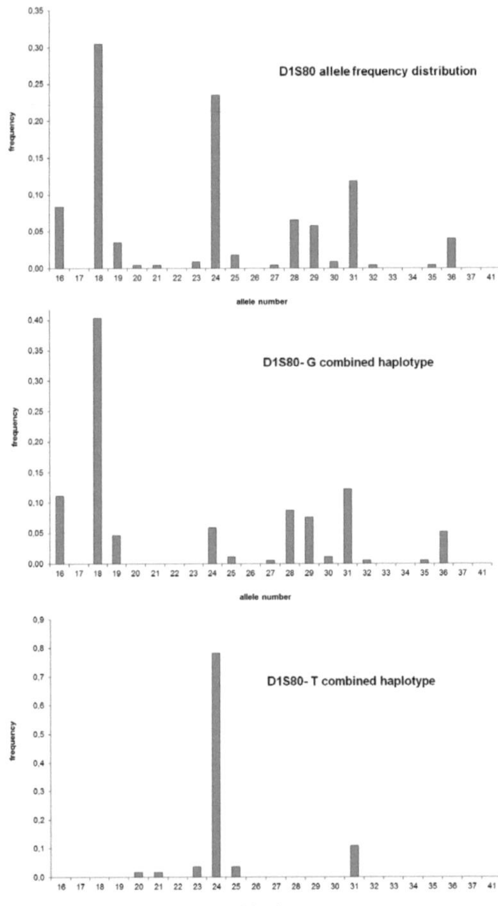

Fig. 8. D1S80 minisatellite allele frequency distributions in Yakut population (Asians).

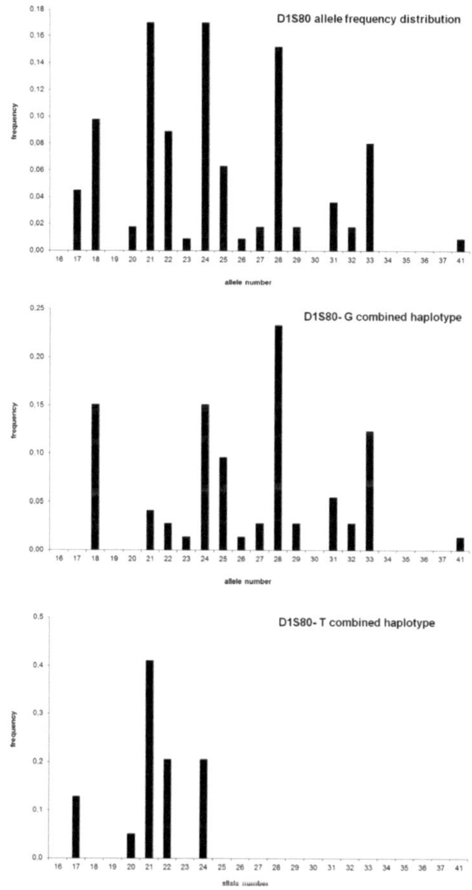

Fig. 9. D1S80 minisatellite allele frequency distributions in Sub-Saharan African population

The allele frequency patterns of the D1S80 locus are multimodal in many different populations (Duncan et al. 1997, Verbenko et al. 2006, Khrunin et al., 2007; Walsh and Eckhoff 2007), and similar patterns were observed in the population samples presented in the current study. However, unlike other studies that did not provide any data on the potential contribution of homoplasy to the allele spectra observed, the use of a system including SNPs allowed us to describe and analyze the distribution patterns of the D1S80 alleles according to their chromosomal location. We started with the analysis of the chromosome-related patterns of D1S80 alleles in samples from Russia (Russians and Yakuts). We paid particular attention to the analysis of D1S80 polymorphisms among northern Russians (individuals from the Mezen district of the Arkhangelsk region), who exhibit differences from other Russians and proximity to the Finno-Ugric- and Baltic-speaking populations (Balanovsky et al. 2008; Khrunin et al. 2009; Limborska et al., 2011b). Yakuts are typical North Asians (Cavalli-Sforza et al. 1996) who are one of the groups that is genetically most distant from Russians (Khrunin et al. 2005, 2007; Verbenko et al., 2005; Flegontova et al., 2009). Subsequently, taking into account the extensive data available on the D1S80 polymorphism among African populations, we compared the D1S80 allele patterns of Russians and Yakuts with our African samples. Although our African DNAs were collected from students who presumably came from all over sub-Saharan Africa, the final distribution of D1S80 allele frequencies observed did not differ significantly from the spectra described for African populations in general (Herrera et al., 2004).

The empirical haplotype phase determination subdivided the total D1S80 allele set into two haploid allele spectra marked with the corresponding alleles of the rs16824398 SNP. In non-African samples, the major D1S80 alleles (18 and 24) were associated with a different SNP background. In the context of this finding, the differences in D1S80 allele spectra between populations of different ethnic origins described previously may be explained by the different ratio of chromosomes with T and G alleles. In our study, these frequencies were close in Russian samples from Smolensk and Mezen, and were different in the Yakut population.

The comparison of D1S80 allele distributions on each of the SNP backgrounds in the populations studied suggests an African origin for both the European and Asian SNP–VNTR haplotypes. In the non-African samples, the most frequent VNTR allele had 24 repeats on chromosomes carrying the T allele and 18 repeats on chromosomes carrying the G allele; the frequencies of these alleles were lower in the African samples. The most frequent alleles in the African samples were VNTR alleles with 21 repeats (on chromosomes with the T allele) and 28 repeats (on chromosomes with the G allele). Generally, the African samples revealed an expanded spectrum of frequent VNTR alleles on both types of chromosomes. This observation is consistent with the corresponding greater values of genetic diversity estimated for Africans.

Our results suggest that, during their migration out of Africa, modern humans carried only a subset of the VNTR spectrum on each of the SNP backgrounds tested. The further evolutionary history of non-African groups (European and Asian ancestors) was accompanied by founding bottlenecks, which were stronger in Asian populations (Keinan et al. 2007, Auton et al. 2009), resulting in the current different ratio of chromosomes with G and T alleles. The greater genetic diversity estimated on the G background for each population suggests that the rs16824398 locus with G at a polymorphic position is a more ancestral sequence than the T-containing variant. This is also consistent with the results of the analysis of corresponding reference sequences in apes, where only G variants are found (the Ensembl project).

Thus, our study demonstrated the effectiveness of applying a haplotyping approach to the analysis of VNTR polymorphisms. Using this method, we identified the chromosome-related characteristics of D1S80 allele patterns, as well as their population features. Taken in the context of other studies, our main findings also illustrate clearly the potential advantages of this SNPrs1682498-D1S80 system over single D1S80 locus testing in population studies and in cases of complex kinship diagnoses.

The subdivision of the D1S80 allele spectrum shape on the linked SNP background is indicative of populations of the main human groups. Considering the SNP ancestral state, the data obtained conform to the out-of-Africa hypothesis of evolution of human populations and provide some details regarding the migration scenario of the main human groups. The application of this SNP–VNTR approach to different sites of the autosomal genome may provide detailed insights into population microevolution.

7. Conclusion

In the past few years, minisatellites have been on the periphery of the attention of researchers. The current focus of interest is the use of SNPs in population studies because of new high-yield methods of testing (DNA microarrays).

Recently, another type of tandemly repeated hypervariable regions of the genome—microsatellites—received renewed interest, as some of them turn out to be the basis of a number of hereditary diseases. This has contributed to the development of new studies of microsatellites, which resulted in certain fundamental conclusions regarding their origin in evolution, the direction of their variability, and their role in the functioning of genomes.

However, existing situation does not negate the significance of minisatellites as very important regions of the genome, especially considering that it has become clear that some of them have a regulatory role regarding the genome. Because of the significant advances in whole-genome sequencing technologies, it can be assumed that, in the near future, the detailed study of minisatellites will be possible as it becomes clear how the features of their appearance and their manner of variability are different from those of microsatellites.

Here, we have tried to show the relevance, importance, and effectiveness of minisatellites based on the example of the use of two minisatellites (D1S80 and 3'*APOB*) in population research. Each of the two minisatellites is located at different chromosomes and can trace the evolutionary trajectory of the population, as it is marked by the corresponding genome segment. It is believed that the genome contains a lot of sites, each of which keeps its own evolutionary history record.

The variability of each of the markers studied (D1S80 and 3'*APOB*) in populations of Eastern Europe agrees quite well with the picture obtained from the analysis of anthropological data, as well as with historical and ethnographic data. Most analyses of other types of DNA markers have yielded similar differentiation patterns for populations of Eastern Europe (for a review see Verbenko & Limborska, 2008; Limborska et al., 2011b). In the case of multidimensional scaling of the matrix of genetic distances for each of the minisatellites studied, Ural populations were located between the European and Asian populations, which is a visual representation of the human origin and diagnostic properties of the markers. The individual features of the 3'*APOB* minisatellite marker include a good population segregation of the Eastern Slavs and Northern Caucasian language families. The use of the minisatellite marker D1S80 together with the main human-group origin/diagnostic features, allows the determination of the specific evolutionary trajectories of individual populations. For example, this marker can be used to distinguish Eastern Slavonic populations from those with stronger expression of the Finno-Ugric component (northern Russian Arkhangelsk region).

The high degree of differentiation of populations based on the variability of the minisatellite markers D1S80 and 3'*APOB* in combination with the method of multidimensional scaling of data processing allows the differentiation of not only distant, but also closely related populations of one ethnic group. Despite the coincidence of main cluster patterns of population differentiation in Eastern Europe detected for each marker, the analysis of individual minisatellite markers can lead to the identification of the specific features of the population. The pattern of variation observed for each minisatellite marker is specific because of the different positions of the markers in the genome. According to Dobzhansky, the action of evolutionary events (mutations and genetic drift, followed by the action of selection) on populations may result in different effects on some parts of the genome, which leaves a trace on the frequency distribution of alleles in the population (Dobzhansky T, 1970). Thus, we can assume that the frequency distribution of the allelic variants of the D1S80 and 3'*APOB* minisatellite loci can be used to characterize certain features of the genetic history of populations. Taking into account the significant differences observed between the frequency distributions of the allelic variants of minisatellite markers among populations of different main human groups and ethnic groups, these markers should be classified as highly differentiated and origin-diagnostic tools.

Special possibilities appeared in evolutionary studies with the simultaneous detection of minisatellites and a flanking SNP. The analysis of these combined haplotypes allows the subdivision of the allele spectrum based on differences in the allelic state of SNPs with decreased mutation rate. Considering the ancestral state of the SNP, these data provide some details regarding the migration scenario of the main human groups. The application of this SNP–VNTR approach to different sites of the autosomal genome may provide detailed insights into population microevolution. It can be assumed that the use of a set of such markers would allow the most informative description of the structure of the gene pool of a particular region, and the identification of the features of the microevolution, origin, and genetic history of its populations.

8. Acknowledgment

The authors are sincerely grateful to all of their colleagues, including the coauthors of publications that provided the basis of this chapter. The work was partially supported by the Ministry of Science and Education of Russian Federation, the Program of support of the leading scientific schools by the President of Russian Federation, programs of Presidium of Russian Academy of Sciences: "Molecular and Cell Biology" and "Fundamental Sciences for Medicine" (subprogram "Human Polymorphism"), and Russian Foundation for Basic Research. We express sincere appreciation to Dr. Denis V. Khokhrin for preparation of this manuscript.

9. References

Ageeva, R.A. (2000). *Where one's kin from? Peoples of Russia: Names and Fates. Explanatory Dictionary*. Academia, ISBN 5-87444-033-X, Moscow

Akhmetova, V.L., Khusainova, R.I., Iur'ev, E.B., Tuktarova, I.A., Petrova, N.V., Makarov, S.V., Kravchuk, O.I., Pai, G.V., Balanovskaia, E.V., Ginter, E.K. & Khusnutdinova, E.K. (2006). Analysis of polymorphism at nine nuclear genome DNA loci in maris. *Genetika*, Vol.42, No.2, (Feb), pp. 256-273, issn 0016-6758

Alekseeva, T.I. (1973). *Ethnogenesis of Eastern Slavs*. (Book in Russian). Moscow State University, Moscow

Amarger, V., Gauguier, D., Yerle, M., Apiou, F., Pinton, P., Giraudeau, F., Monfouilloux, S., Lathrop, M., Dutrillaux, B., Buard, J. & Vergnaud, G. (1998). Analysis of distribution in the human, pig, and rat genomes points toward a general subtelomeric origin of minisatellite structures. *Genomics*, Vol.52, No.1, (Aug 15), pp. 62-71, issn 0888-7543

Auton, A., Bryc, K., Boyko, A.R., Lohmueller, K.E., Novembre, J., Reynolds, A., Indap, A., Wright, M.H., Degenhardt, J.D., Gutenkunst, R.N., King, K.S., Nelson, M.R. & Bustamante, C.D. (2009). Global distribution of genomic diversity underscores rich complex history of continental human populations. *Genome Res*, Vol.19, No.5, (May), pp. 795-803, issn 1088-9051

Babushkina, N.P. & Kucher, A.N. Functional role of VNTR polymorphism of human genes. *Genetika*, Vol.47, No.6, (Jun), pp. 725-734, issn 0016-6758

Balanovsky, O., Rootsi, S., Pshenichnov, A., Kivisild, T., Churnosov, M., Evseeva, I., Pocheshkhova, E., Boldyreva, M., Yankovsky, N., Balanovska, E. & Villems, R. (2008). Two sources of the Russian patrilineal heritage in their Eurasian context. *Am J Hum Genet*, Vol.82, No.1, (Jan), pp. 236-250, issn 1537-6605 (Electronic)

Barysheva, E.V., Prosniak, M.I., Vlasov, M.S., Golubtsov, V.I., Revazov, A.A., Limborskaia, S.A. & Ginter, E.K. (1989). The use of DNA from phage M13 for the analysis of interindividual polymorphism of human DNA as demonstrated by a population study in Krasnodar city. *Genetika*, Vol.25, No.11, (Nov), pp. 2079-2082, issn 0016-6758

Barysheva, E.V., Bukina, A.M., Petrova, N.V., Limborskaia, S.A. & Ginter, E.K. (1991). Use of DNA polymorphism detected by M13 phage DNA in population studies. *Genetika*, Vol.27, No.3, (Mar), pp. 399-403, issn 0016-6758

Barysheva, E.V., Bukina, A.M., Limborskaia, S.A. & Ginter, E.K. (1991). Analysis of genetic distances between populations using human DNA "fingerprints" detected by a phage M13 DNA probe. *Genetika*, Vol.27, No.9, (Sep), pp. 1493-1498, issn 0016-6758

Bell, G.I., Selby, M.J. & Rutter, W.J. (1982). The highly polymorphic region near the human insulin gene is composed of simple tandemly repeating sequences. *Nature*, Vol.295, No.5844, (Jan 7), pp. 31-35, issn 0028-0836

Belyaeva, O.V., Balanovsky, O.P., Ashworth, L.K., Lebedev, Y.B., Spitsyn, V.A., Guseva, N.A., Erdes, S., Mikulich, A.I., Khusnutdinova, E.K. & Limborska, S.A. (1999). Fine mapping of a polymorphic CA repeat marker on human chromosome 19 and its use in population studies. *Gene*, Vol.230, No.2, (Apr 16), pp. 259-266, issn 0378-1119

Belyaeva, O., Bermisheva, M., Khrunin, A., Slominsky, P., Bebyakova, N., Khusnutdinova, E., Mikulich, A. & Limborska, S. (2003). Mitochondrial DNA variations in Russian and Belorussian populations. *Hum Biol*, Vol.75, No.5, (Oct), pp. 647-660, issn 0018-7143

Bennett, S.T., Lucassen, A.M., Gough, S.C., Powell, E.E., Undlien, D.E., Pritchard, L.E., Merriman, M.E., Kawaguchi, Y., Dronsfield, M.J., Pociot, F. & et al. (1995). Susceptibility to human type 1 diabetes at IDDM2 is determined by tandem repeat variation at the insulin gene minisatellite locus. *Nat Genet*, Vol.9, No.3, (Mar), pp. 284-292, issn 1061-4036

Bermisheva, M.A., Viktorova, T.V., Beliaeva, O., Limborskaia, S.A. & Khusnutdinova, E.K. (2001). Polymorphism of hypervariable segment I of mitochondrial DNA in three ethnic groups of the Volga-Ural region. *Genetika*, Vol.37, No.8, (Aug), pp. 1118-1124, issn 0016-6758

Bermisheva, M.A., Viktorova, T.V. & Khusnutdinova, E.K. (2003). Polymorphism of human mitochondrial DNA. *Genetika*, Vol.39, No.8, (Aug), pp. 1013-1025, issn 0016-6758

Bermisheva, M.A., Petrova, N.V., Zinchenko, R.A., Timkovskaia, E.E., Malyshev, P., Gavrilina, S.G., Ginter, E.K. & Kusnutdinova, E.K. (2007). Population study of the Udmurt population: analysis of ten polymorphic DNA loci of the nuclear genome. *Genetika*, Vol.43, No.5, (May), pp. 688-705, issn 0016-6758

Boerwinkle, E., Xiong, W.J., Fourest, E. & Chan, L. (1989). Rapid typing of tandemly repeated hypervariable loci by the polymerase chain reaction: application to the apolipoprotein B 3' hypervariable region. *Proc Natl Acad Sci U S A*, Vol.86, No.1, (Jan), pp. 212-216, issn 0027-8424

Bois, P. & Jeffreys, A.J. (1999). Minisatellite instability and germline mutation. *Cell Mol Life Sci*, Vol.55, No.12, (Sep), pp. 1636-1648, issn 1420-682X

Bois, P.R. (2003). Hypermutable minisatellites, a human affair? *Genomics*, Vol.81, No.4, (Apr), pp. 349-355, issn 0888-7543

Buard, J. & Vergnaud, G. (1994). Complex recombination events at the hypermutable minisatellite CEB1 (D2S90). *EMBO J*, Vol.13, No.13, (Jul 1), pp. 3203-3210, issn 0261-4189

Budowle, B., Chakraborty, R., Giusti, A.M., Eisenberg, A.J. & Allen, R.C. (1991). Analysis of the VNTR locus D1S80 by the PCR followed by high-resolution PAGE. *Am J Hum Genet*, Vol.48, No.1, (Jan), pp. 137-144, issn 0002-9297

Budowle, B., Baechtel, F.S., Smerick, J.B., Presley, K.W., Giusti, A.M., Parsons, G., Alevy, M.C. & Chakraborty, R. (1995). D1S80 population data in African Americans, Caucasians, southeastern Hispanics, southwestern Hispanics, and Orientals. *J Forensic Sci*, Vol.40, No.1, (Jan), pp. 38-44, issn 0022-1198

Bunak, V.V. (1965). *Origin and Ethnic History of the Russian Nation. (Proiskhozhdeniye i etnicheskaya istoriya russkogo naroda),* Nauka, Moscow.

Buresi, C., Desmarais, E., Vigneron, S., Lamarti, H., Smaoui, N., Cambien, F. & Roizes, G. (1996). Structural analysis of the minisatellite present at the 3' end of the human apolipoprotein B gene: new definition of the alleles and evolutionary implications. *Hum Mol Genet*, Vol.5, No.1, (Jan), pp. 61-68, issn 0964-6906

Capon, D.J., Chen, E.Y., Levinson, A.D., Seeburg, P.H. & Goeddel, D.V. (1983). Complete nucleotide sequences of the T24 human bladder carcinoma oncogene and its normal homologue. *Nature*, Vol.302, No.5903, (Mar 3), pp. 33-37, issn 0028-0836

Cavalli-Sforza, L.L. & Feldman, M.W. (2003). The application of molecular genetic approaches to the study of human evolution. *Nat Genet*, Vol.33 Suppl, (Mar), pp. 266-275, issn 1061-4036

Chen, B., Guo, Z., He, P., Ye, P., Buresi, C. & Roizes, G. (1999). Structure and function of alleles in the 3' end region of human apoB gene. *Chin Med J (Engl)*, Vol.112, No.3, (Mar), pp. 221-223, issn 0366-6999

Chistiakov, D.A., Gavrilov, D.K., Ovchinnikov, I.V. & Nosikov, V.V. (1993). Analysis of the distribution of alleles of four hypervariable tandem repeats among unrelated Russian individuals living in Moscow, using the polymerase chain reaction. *Mol Biol (Mosk)*, Vol.27, No.6, (Nov-Dec), pp. 1304-1314, issn 0026-8984

Choong, M.L., Koay, E.S., Khaw, M.C. & Aw, T.C. (1999). Apolipoprotein B 5'-Ins/Del and 3'-VNTR polymorphisms in Chinese, malay and Indian singaporeans. *Hum Hered*, Vol.49, No.1, (Jan), pp. 31-40, issn 0001-5652

Das, K. & Mastana, S.S. (2003). Genetic variation at three VNTR loci in three tribal populations of Orissa, India. *Ann Hum Biol*, Vol.30, No.3, (May-Jun), pp. 237-249, issn 0301-4460

Deka, R., Chakraborty, R., DeCroo, S., Rothhammer, F., Barton, S.A. & Ferrell, R.E. (1992). Characteristics of polymorphism at a VNTR locus 3' to the apolipoprotein B gene in five human populations. *Am J Hum Genet*, Vol.51, No.6, (Dec), pp. 1325-1333, issn 0002-9297

Destro-Bisol, G., Capelli, C. & Belledi, M. (2000). Inferring microevolutionary patterns from allele-size frequency distributions of minisatellite loci: a worldwide study of the APOB 3' hypervariable region polymorphism. *Hum Biol*, Vol.72, No.5, (Oct), pp. 733-751, issn 0018-7143

Dobzhansky, T. (1970). *Genetics of the Evolutionary Process*, Columbia Univ. Press, ISBN-13: 978-0231083065 , New York.

Duncan, G., Thomas, E., Gallo, J.C., Baird, L.S., Garrison, J. & Herrera, R.J. (1996). Human phylogenetic relationships according to the D1S80 locus. *Genetica*, Vol.98, No.3, pp. 277-287, issn 0016-6707

Dzhincharadze, A.G., Ivanov, P.L. & Ryskov, A.P. (1987). Genome "dactyloscopy". Characteristics of the human cloned sequence JIN 600 in vector M13 with properties of highly polymorphic DNA marker. *Dokl Akad Nauk SSSR*, Vol.295, No.1, (Jul-Aug), pp. 230-233, issn 0002-3264

Flegontova, O.V., Khrunin, A.V., Lylova, O.I., Tarskaia, L.A., Spitsyn, V.A., Mikulich, A.I. & Limborska, S.A. (2009). Haplotype frequencies at the DRD2 locus in populations of the East European Plain. *BMC Genet*, Vol.10, pp. 62, issn 1471-2156 (Electronic)

Fuke, S., Suo, S., Takahashi, N., Koike, H., Sasagawa, N. & Ishiura, S. (2001). The VNTR polymorphism of the human dopamine transporter (DAT1) gene affects gene expression. *Pharmacogenomics J*, Vol.1, No.2, pp. 152-156, issn 1470-269X

Gemayel, R., Vinces, M.D., Legendre, M. & Verstrepen, K.J. Variable tandem repeats accelerate evolution of coding and regulatory sequences. *Annu Rev Genet*, Vol.44, pp. 445-477, issn 1545-2948

Harris, R.F. (2002). Hapmap flap. *Curr Biol*, Vol.12, No.24, (Dec 23), pp. R827, issn 0960-9822

Herrera, R.J., Adrien, L.R., Ruiz, L.M., Sanabria, N.Y. & Duncan, G. (2004). D1S80 single-locus discrimination among African populations. *Hum Biol*, Vol.76, No.1, (Feb), pp. 87-108, issn 0018-7143

Hong-Sheng, G., Peng, Z., Cheng-Bo, Y. & Sheng-Bin, L. (2009). HGD-Chn: The Database of Genome Diversity and Variation for Chinese Populations. *Leg Med (Tokyo)*, Vol.11 Suppl 1, (Apr), pp. S201-202, issn 1873-4162 (Electronic)

Huang, L.S. & Breslow, J.L. (1987). A unique AT-rich hypervariable minisatellite 3' to the ApoB gene defines a high information restriction fragment length polymorphism. *J Biol Chem*, Vol.262, No.19, (Jul 5), pp. 8952-8955, issn 0021-9258

Jeffreys, A.J., Wilson, V. & Thein, S.L. (1985). Hypervariable 'minisatellite' regions in human DNA. *Nature*, Vol.314, No.6006, (Mar 7-13), pp. 67-73, issn 0028-0836

Jeffreys, A.J., Wilson, V., Neumann, R. & Keyte, J. (1988). Amplification of human minisatellites by the polymerase chain reaction: towards DNA fingerprinting of single cells. *Nucleic Acids Res*, Vol.16, No.23, (Dec 9), pp. 10953-10971, issn 0305-1048

Jeffreys, A.J., Tamaki, K., MacLeod, A., Monckton, D.G., Neil, D.L. & Armour, J.A. (1994). Complex gene conversion events in germline mutation at human minisatellites. *Nat Genet*, Vol.6, No.2, (Feb), pp. 136-145, issn 1061-4036

Jurka, J. & Gentles, A.J. (2006). Origin and diversification of minisatellites derived from human Alu sequences. *Gene*, Vol.365, (Jan 3), pp. 21-26, issn 0378-1119

Kalnin, V.V., Kalnina, O.V., Prosniak, M.I., Khidiatova, I.M., Khusnutdinova, E.K., Raphicov, K.S., Limborska, S.A. (1995). Use of DNA fingerprinting for human population genetic studies, Vol. 247, No. 4, (May 20), pp. 488-93.

Kawakami, K., Salonga, D., Park, J.M., Danenberg, K.D., Uetake, H., Brabender, J., Omura, K., Watanabe, G. & Danenberg, P.V. (2001). Different lengths of a polymorphic repeat sequence in the thymidylate synthase gene affect translational efficiency but not its gene expression. *Clin Cancer Res*, Vol.7, No.12, (Dec), pp. 4096-4101, issn 1078-0432

Keinan, A., Mullikin, J.C., Patterson, N. & Reich, D. (2007). Measurement of the human allele frequency spectrum demonstrates greater genetic drift in East Asians than in Europeans. *Nat Genet*, Vol.39, No.10, (Oct), pp. 1251-1255, issn 1546-1718 (Electronic)

Kelkar, Y.D., Tyekucheva, S., Chiaromonte, F. & Makova, K.D. (2008). The genome-wide determinants of human and chimpanzee microsatellite evolution. *Genome Res*, Vol.18, No.1, (Jan), pp. 30-38, issn 1088-9051

Kendrew J.C., Lawrence E.L.(1994) *The encyclopedia of molecular biology. Blackwell Science*, ISBN 0-632-02182-9, Oxford

Khar'kov, V.N., Stepanov, V.A., Borinskaia, S.A., Kozhekbaeva Zh, M., Gusar, V.A., Grechanina, E., Puzyrev, V.P., Khusnutdinova, E.K. & Iankovskii, N.K. (2004). Structure of the gene pool of eastern Ukrainians from Y-chromosome haplogroups. *Genetika*, Vol.40, No.3, (Mar), pp. 415-421, issn 0016-6758

Khrunin, A., Mihailov, E., Nikopensius, T., Krjutskov, K., Limborska, S. & Metspalu, A. (2009). Analysis of allele and haplotype diversity across 25 genomic regions in three Eastern European populations. *Hum Hered*, Vol.68, No.1, pp. 35-44, issn 1423-0062 (Electronic)

Khrunin, A.V., Bebiakova, N.A., Ivanov, V.P., Solodilova, M.A. & Limborskaia, S.A. (2005). Polymorphism of Y-chromosomal microsatellites in Russian populations from the northern and southern Russia as exemplified by the populations of Kursk and Arkhangel'sk Oblast. *Genetika*, Vol.41, No.8, (Aug), pp. 1125-1131, issn 0016-6758

Khusnutdinova, E.K., Viktorova, T.V., Fatkhlislamova, R.I. & Galeeva, A.R. (1999). Evaluation of the relative contribution of Caucasoid and Mongoloid components in the formation of ethnic groups of the Volga-Ural region according to data of DNA polymorphism. *Genetika*, Vol.35, No.8, (Aug), pp. 1132-1137, issn 0016-6758

Khusnutdinova, E.K., Viktorova, T.V., Akhmetova, V.L., Mustafina, O.E., Fatkhlislamova, R.I., Balanovskaia, E.V., Petrova, N.V., Makarov, S.V., Kravchuk, O.I., Pai, G.V. & Ginter, E.K. (2003). Population-genetic structure of Chuvashia (from data on eight DNA loci in the nuclear genome). *Genetika*, Vol.39, No.11, (Nov), pp. 1550-1563, issn 0016-6758

Klenova, E., Scott, A.C., Roberts, J., Shamsuddin, S., Lovejoy, E.A., Bergmann, S., Bubb, V.J., Royer, H.D. & Quinn, J.P. (2004). YB-1 and CTCF differentially regulate the 5-HTT polymorphic intron 2 enhancer which predisposes to a variety of neurological disorders. *J Neurosci*, Vol.24, No.26, (Jun 30), pp. 5966-5973, issn 1529-2401 (Electronic)

Kravchenko, S.A., Maliarchuk, O.S. & Livshits, L.A. (1996). A population genetics study of the allelic polymorphism in the hypervariable region of the apolipoprotein B gene in the population of different regions of Ukraine. *Tsitol Genet*, Vol.30, No.5, (Sep-Oct), pp. 35-41, issn 0564-3783

Kravchenko, S.A., Slominskii, P.A., Bets, L.A., Stepanova, A.V., Mikulich, A.I., Limborskaia, S.A. & Livshits, L.A. (2002). Polymorphism of the STR-locus of Y chromosomes in Eastern Slavs in three populations from Belorussia, Russia and the Ukraine. *Genetika*, Vol.38, No.1, (Jan), pp. 97-104, issn 0016-6758

Kravchenko, S.A., Malyarchuk, S.G. & Pampukha, V.M. (2001). *Genetika i selektziya na Ukraine na rubezhe tysyacheletiy (Genetics and Selection in the Ukraine at the Boundary of Millennia)*, Vol. 4, pp. 410–422, Logos, Kiev

Kuzeev, R.G. (1985). Peoples of Povolzhye and Priuralye. (Narody Povolzhya i Priuralya), Nauka, Moscow.

Lahermo, P., Sajantila, A., Sistonen, P., Lukka, M., Aula, P., Peltonen, L. & Savontaus, M.L. (1996). The genetic relationship between the Finns and the Finnish Saami (Lapps): analysis of nuclear DNA and mtDNA. *Am J Hum Genet*, Vol.58, No.6, (Jun), pp. 1309-1322, issn 0002-9297

Latorra, D., Stern, C.M. & Schanfield, M.S. (1994). Characterization of human AFLP systems apolipoprotein B, phenylalanine hydroxylase, and D1S80. *PCR Methods Appl*, Vol.3, No.6, (Jun), pp. 351-358, issn 1054-9803

Levinson, G. & Gutman, G.A. (1987). Slipped-strand mispairing: a major mechanism for DNA sequence evolution. *Mol Biol Evol*, Vol.4, No.3, (May), pp. 203-221, issn 0737-4038

Lewis, P.O., Zaykin, D. (2001). *Genetic Data Analysis: Computer program for the analysis of allelic data. Version 1.0 (d16c).* Available from: http://lewis.eeb.uconn.edu/lewishome/software.html

Limborska, S.A., Khrunin, A.V., Flegontova, O.V., Tasitz, V.A. & Verbenko, D.A. (2011a). Specificity of genetic diversity in D1S80 revealed by SNP-VNTR haplotyping. *Ann Hum Biol*, Vol.38, No.5, (Sep), pp. 564-569, issn 1464-5033 (Electronic)

Limborska, S.A., Verbenko, D.A., Khrunin, A.V., Slominsky, P.A., Bebyakova, N.A. (2011b) Ethnic genomics: analysis of genome polymorphism of Archangelsk region. *Bulletin of Moscow University.Series XXIII. Anthropology, No.3*, pp. 100-119, ISSN 0201–7385

Ludwig, E.H., Friedl, W. & McCarthy, B.J. (1989). High-resolution analysis of a hypervariable region in the human apolipoprotein B gene. *Am J Hum Genet*, Vol.45, No.3, (Sep), pp. 458-464, issn 0002-9297

Malyarchuk, B.A. & Derenko, M.V. (2001). Mitochondrial DNA variability in Russians and Ukrainians: implication to the origin of the Eastern Slavs. *Ann Hum Genet*, Vol.65, No.Pt 1, (Jan), pp. 63-78, issn 0003-4800

Malyarchuk, B.A., Grzybowski, T., Derenko, M.V., Czarny, J., Wozniak, M. & Miscicka-Sliwka, D. (2002). Mitochondrial DNA variability in Poles and Russians. *Ann Hum Genet*, Vol.66, No.Pt 4, (Jul), pp. 261-283, issn 0003-4800

Marz, W., Ruzicka, V., Fisher, E., Russ, A.P., Schneider, W. & Gross, W. (1993). Typing of the 3' hypervariable region of the apolipoprotein B gene: approaches, pitfalls, and applications. *Electrophoresis*, Vol.14, No.3, (Mar), pp. 169-173, issn 0173-0835

Mastana, S.S. & Papiha, S.S. (2001). D1S80 distribution in world populations with new data from the UK and the Indian sub-continent. *Ann Hum Biol*, Vol.28, No.3, (May-Jun), pp. 308-318, issn 0301-4460

Miklos, G.L. & John, B. (1979). Heterochromatin and satellite DNA in man: properties and prospects. *Am J Hum Genet*, Vol.31, No.3, (May), pp. 264-280, issn 0002-9297

Miller, MP. (1997). *R by C: A program that performs Fisher's Exact test on any sized contingency table through the use of the Metropolis algorithm*, Available from: http://bioweb.usu.edu/mpmbio/

Mirabal, S., Regueiro, M., Cadenas, A.M., Cavalli-Sforza, L.L., Underhill, P.A., Verbenko, D.A., Limborska, S.A. & Herrera, R.J. (2009). Y-chromosome distribution within the geo-linguistic landscape of northwestern Russia. *Eur J Hum Genet*, Vol.17, No.10, (Oct), pp. 1260-1273, issn 1476-5438 (Electronic)

Nakahara, M., Shimozawa, M., Nakamura, Y., Irino, Y., Morita, M., Kudo, Y. & Fukami, K. (2005). A novel phospholipase C, PLC(eta)2, is a neuron-specific isozyme. *J Biol Chem*, Vol.280, No.32, (Aug 12), pp. 29128-29134, issn 0021-9258

Nakamura, Y., Carlson, M., Krapcho, K. & White, R. (1988). Isolation and mapping of a polymorphic DNA sequence (pMCT118) on chromosome 1p D1S80. *Nucleic Acids Res*, Vol.16, No.19, (Oct 11), pp. 9364, issn 0305-1048

Nei, M. (1972). Genetic Distance between Populations. *The American Naturalist*, Vol.106, No.949, pp. 283-292

Orekhov, V., Poltoraus, A., Zhivotovsky, L.A., Spitsyn, V., Ivanov, P. & Yankovsky, N. (1999). Mitochondrial DNA sequence diversity in Russians. *FEBS Lett*, Vol.445, No.1, (Feb 19), pp. 197-201, issn 0014-5793

Paquette, J., Giannoukakis, N., Polychronakos, C., Vafiadis, P. & Deal, C. (1998). The INS 5' variable number of tandem repeats is associated with IGF2 expression in humans. *J Biol Chem*, Vol.273, No.23, (Jun 5), pp. 14158-14164, issn 0021-9258

Pena, S.D. & Chakraborty, R. (1994). Paternity testing in the DNA era. *Trends Genet*, Vol.10, No.6, (Jun), pp. 204-209, issn 0168-9525

Poltl, R., Luckenbach, C., Reinhold, J., Fimmers, R. & Ritter, H. (1996). Comparison of German population data on the apoB-HVR locus with other Caucasian, Asian and black populations. *Forensic Sci Int*, Vol.80, No.3, (Jul 12), pp. 221-227, issn 0379-0738

Popova, S.N., Mikulich, A.I., Slominskii, P.A., Shadrina, M.I., Pomazanova, M.A. & Limborskaia, S.A. (1999). Polymorphism of the (CTG)n repeat in the myotonin protein kinase (DM) gene in Belarussian populations: analysis of interethnic heterogeneity. *Genetika*, Vol.35, No.7, (Jul), pp. 994-997, issn 0016-6758

Popova, S.N., Slominsky, P.A., Pocheshnova, E.A., Balanovskaya, E.V., Tarskaya, L.A., Bebyakova, N.A., Bets, L.V., Ivanov, V.P., Livshits, L.A., Khusnutdinova, E.K., Spitcyn, V.A. & Limborska, S.A. (2001). Polymorphism of trinucleotide repeats in loci DM, DRPLA and SCA1 in East European populations. *Eur J Hum Genet*, Vol.9, No.11, (Nov), pp. 829-835, issn 1018-4813

Popova, S.N., Slominskii, P.A., Galushkin, S.N., Tarskaia, L.A., Spitsyn, V.A., Guseva, I.A. & Limborskaia, S.A. (2002). Analysis of the allele polymorphism of (CTG)n and (GAG)n triplet repeats in DM, DRPLA, and SCA1 genes in various populations of Russia. *Genetika*, Vol.38, No.11, (Nov), pp. 1549-1553, issn 0016-6758

Proudfoot, N.J., Gil, A. & Maniatis, T. (1982). The structure of the human zeta-globin gene and a closely linked, nearly identical pseudogene. *Cell*, Vol.31, No.3 Pt 2, (Dec), pp. 553-563, issn 0092-8674

Renges, H.H., Peacock, R., Dunning, A.M., Talmud, P. & Humphries, S.E. (1992). Genetic relationship between the 3'-VNTR and diallelic apolipoprotein B gene polymorphisms: haplotype analysis in individuals of European and south Asian origin. *Ann Hum Genet*, Vol.56, No.Pt 1, (Jan), pp. 11-33, issn 0003-4800

Ryskov, A.P., Tokarskaia, O.N., Verbovaia, L.V., Dzhincharadze, A.G. & Gintsburg, A.L. (1988). Genomic fingerprinting of microorganisms: its use as a hybridization probe of phage M13 DNA. *Genetika*, Vol.24, No.7, (Jul), pp. 1310-1313, issn 0016-6758

Ryskov, A.P., Faizov, T., Alimov, A.M. & Romanova, E.A. (1990). Genomic fingerprinting: new possibilities in determining the species identity of Brucella. *Genetika*, Vol.26, No.1, (Jan), pp. 130-133, issn 0016-6758

Sajantila, A., Budowle, B., Strom, M., Johnsson, V., Lukka, M., Peltonen, L. & Ehnholm, C. (1992). PCR amplification of alleles at the DIS80 locus: comparison of a Finnish and a North American Caucasian population sample, and forensic casework evaluation. *Am J Hum Genet*, Vol.50, No.4, (Apr), pp. 816-825, issn 0002-9297

Sajantila, A., Lukka, M. & Syvanen, A.C. (1999). Experimentally observed germline mutations at human micro- and minisatellite loci. *Eur J Hum Genet*, Vol.7, No.2, (Feb-Mar), pp. 263-266, issn 1018-4813

Schlotterer, C. (1998). Microsatellites, In: *Molecular genetics analysis of populations*, Hoelzel, A.R., pp. 237 , IRL Press, Oxford Univ. Press, ISBN 9780199636358 , London

Sedov, V.V. (1979). *Origin and early history of Slavs* (Book in Russian). Nauka, Moscow

Semenova, S.K., Romanova, E.A. & Ryskov, A.P. (1996). Genetic differentiation of helminths on the basis of data of polymerase chain reaction using random primers. *Genetika*, Vol.32, No.2, (Feb), pp. 304-309, issn 0016-6758

Semina, E.V., Bukina, A.M., Startseva, E.A., Limborskaia, S.A. & Ginter, E.K. (1993). Genetic distances between various ethnic populations calculated on the basis of polymorphism of DNA detected by the hypervariable phage M13 DNA probe. *Genetika*, Vol.29, No.10, (Oct), pp. 1612-1619, issn 0016-6758

Shabrova, E.V., Khusnutdinova, E.K., Tarskaia, L.A., Mikulich, A.I., Abolmasov, N.N. & Limborska, S.A. (2004). DNA diversity of human populations from Eastern Europe and Siberia studied by multilocus DNA fingerprinting. *Mol Genet Genomics*, Vol.271, No.3, (Apr), pp. 291-297, issn 1617-4615

Shabrova, E.V., Limborska, S.A. & Ryskov, A.P. (2006). Multilocus DNA fingerprinting-genotyping based on micro and minisatellite polymorphisms, *In: Focus on DNA fingerprinting research*, Read, M.M. Nova Publishers, ISBN 9781594549533, New York.

Song, J., Yoon, Y., Park, K.U., Park, J., Hong, Y.J., Hong, S.H. & Kim, J.Q. (2003). Genotype-specific influence on nitric oxide synthase gene expression, protein concentrations, and enzyme activity in cultured human endothelial cells. *Clin Chem*, Vol.49, No.6 Pt 1, (Jun), pp. 847-852, issn 0009-9147

Spitsyn, V.A., Khorte, M.V., Pogoda, T.V., Slominsky, P.A., Nurbaev, S.D., Agapova, R.K. & Limborska, S.A. (2000). Apolipoprotein B 3'-VNTR polymorphism in the Udmurt population. *Hum Hered*, Vol.50, No.4, (Jul-Aug), pp. 224-226, issn 0001-5652

Stepanov, V.A., Spiridonova, M.G. & Puzyrev, V.P. (2003). Comparative phylogenetic study of native north Eurasian populations from a panel of autosomal microsatellite loci. *Genetika*, Vol.39, No.11, (Nov), pp. 1564-1572, issn 0016-6758

Tanaka, T. (2005). International HapMap project. *Nihon Rinsho*, Vol.63 Suppl 12, (Dec), pp. 29-34, issn 0047-1852

Vassart, G., Georges, M., Monsieur, R., Brocas, H., Lequarre, A.S. & Christophe, D. (1987). A sequence in M13 phage detects hypervariable minisatellites in human and animal DNA. *Science*, Vol.235, No.4789, (Feb 6), pp. 683-684, issn 0036-8075

Verbenko, D.A., Pogoda, T.V., Spitsyn, V.A., Mikulich, A.I., Bets, L.V., Bebyakova, N.A., Ivanov, V.P., Abolmasov, N.N., Pocheshkhova, E.A., Balanovskaya, E.V., Tarskaya,

L.A., Sorensen, M.V. & Limborska, S.A. (2003). Apolipoprotein B 3'-VNTR polymorphism in Eastern European populations. *Eur J Hum Genet*, Vol.11, No.6, (Jun), pp. 444-451, issn 1018-4813

Verbenko, D.A., Kekeeva, T.V., Pogoda, T.V., Khusnutdinova, E.K., Mikulich, A.I., Kravchenko, S.A., Livshits, L.A., Bebyakova, N.A. & Limborska, S.A. (2003). Allele frequencies for D1S80 (pMCT118) locus in some East European populations. *J Forensic Sci*, Vol.48, No.1, (Jan), pp. 207-208, issn 0022-1198

Verbenko, D.A., Pocheshkhova, E.A., Balanovskaya, E.V., Marshanija, E.Z., Kvitzinija, P.K. & Limborska, S.A. (2004). Polymorphisms of D1 S80 and 3'ApoB minisatellite loci in Northern Caucasus populations. *J Forensic Sci*, Vol.49, No.1, (Jan), pp. 178-180, issn 0022-1198

Verbenko, D.A., Knjazev, A.N., Mikulich, A.I., Khusnutdinova, E.K., Bebyakova, N.A. & Limborska, S.A. (2005). Variability of the 3'APOB minisatellite locus in Eastern Slavonic populations. *Hum Hered*, Vol.60, No.1, pp. 10-18, issn 0001-5652

Verbenko, D.A., Slominsky, P.A., Spitsyn, V.A., Bebyakova, N.A., Khusnutdinova, E.K., Mikulich, A.I., Tarskaia, L.A., Sorensen, M.V., Ivanov, V.P., Bets, L.V. & Limborska, S.A. (2006). Polymorphisms at locus D1S80 and other hypervariable regions in the analysis of Eastern European ethnic group relationships. *Ann Hum Biol*, Vol.33, No.5-6, (Sep-Dec), pp. 570-584, issn 0301-4460

Verbenko, D.A., Limborskaia, S.A. (2008). Human minisatellite markers: D1S80 locus in population studies. *Mol Gen Mikrobiol Virusol*, No. 2, pp. 3-11.

Vergnaud, G. & Denoeud, F. (2000). Minisatellites: mutability and genome architecture. *Genome Res*, Vol.10, No.7, (Jul), pp. 899-907, issn 1088-9051

Verstrepen, K.J., Jansen, A., Lewitter, F. & Fink, G.R. (2005). Intragenic tandem repeats generate functional variability. *Nat Genet*, Vol.37, No.9, (Sep), pp. 986-990, issn 1061-4036

Walsh, S.J. & Eckhoff, C. (2007). Australian Aboriginal population genetics at the D1S80 VNTR locus. *Ann Hum Biol*, Vol.34, No.5, (Sep-Oct), pp. 557-565, issn 0301-4460

Watanabe, G. & Shimizu, K. (2002). DNA sequence analysis of long PCR amplified products at the D1S80 locus. *Leg Med (Tokyo)*, Vol.4, No.1, (Mar), pp. 37-39, issn 1344-6223

Weir, B.S. (1996). *Genetic data analysis* (1st), Sinauer Associates, Inc, ISBN 0878939075, Sunderland

Weller, P., Jeffreys, A.J., Wilson, V. & Blanchetot, A. (1984). Organization of the human myoglobin gene. *EMBO J*, Vol.3, No.2, (Feb), pp. 439-446, issn 0261-4189

Wyman, A.R. & White, R. (1980). A highly polymorphic locus in human DNA. *Proc Natl Acad Sci U S A*, Vol.77, No.11, (Nov), pp. 6754-6758, issn 0027-8424

Yeh, FC, Yang, R-C & Boyle, T. (1999) *POPGENE version 1.32*, Available from: http://www.ualberta.ca/~fyeh/

Zago, M.A., Silva Junior, W.A., Tavella, M.H., Santos, S.E., Guerreiro, J.F. & Figueiredo, M.S. (1996). Interpopulational and intrapopulational genetic diversity of Amerindians as revealed by six variable number of tandem repeats. *Hum Hered*, Vol.46, No.5, (Sep-Oct), pp. 274-289, issn 0001-5652

Zhang, M.X., Ou, H., Shen, Y.H., Wang, J., Coselli, J. & Wang, X.L. (2005). Regulation of endothelial nitric oxide synthase by small RNA. *Proc Natl Acad Sci U S A*, Vol.102, No.47, (Nov 22), pp. 16967-16972, issn 0027-8424

Zhivotovskii, L.A. (2006). Population aspects of forensic genetics. *Genetika*, Vol.42, No.10, (Oct), pp. 1426-1436, issn 0016-6758

5

Polymorphism

Oliver Mayo
CSIRO Livestock Industries, Adelaide
Australia

1. Introduction

"I refer to those genera which have sometimes been called 'protean' or 'polymorphic,' in which the species present an inordinate amount of variation; and hardly two naturalists can agree which forms to rank as species and which as varieties. ... I am inclined to suspect that we see in these polymorphic genera variations in points of structure which are of no service or disservice to the species, and which consequently have not been seized on and rendered definite by natural selection, as hereafter will be explained." (Darwin 1859 Ch. 2) Although Darwin was pointing to taxonomic problems caused by meaningless variation here, he clearly understood that a species could manifest variations that were neutral in the face of natural selection, and hence were not removed by natural selection. With no explicit demographic or genetical model, Darwin could not take the discussion further, but the concept of polymorphic variation within a species is clearly 150 years old at least.

Once genetics had been set on a sound footing by Mendel and his rediscoverers, genetic polymorphisms were rapidly identified. Sex determination was one of the first and most important; other outbreeding mechanisms, such as heteromorphic self-incompatibility, a major subject of Darwin's own research, were soon identified as functional polymorphisms.

Polymorphism was thus identified as variability that was genetically determined. How it related to other phenotypic variability was not clear. At the time when Mendelian genetics and statistically measured quantitative genetic variation were reconciled by Fisher (1918), the role of individual genes in influencing quantitative variation was barely initiated, through the study of, for example, dwarfing genes.

2. Balanced polymorphism

"If selection favours the homozygotes, no stable equilibrium will be possible, and selection will then tend to eliminate whichever gene is below its equilibrium proportion; such factors will therefore not commonly be found in nature: if, on the other hand, the selection favours the heterozygote, there is a condition of stable equilibrium, and the factor will continue in the stock. Such factors should therefore be commonly found, and may explain instances of hybrid vigour, and to some extent the deleterious effects sometimes brought about by inbreeding." (Fisher 1922 p. 324)

The argument, which introduces notation etc., is as follows. Consider a diallelic locus with two alleles, A_1 and A_2, having frequencies p and q in an indefinitely large population with random mating. Then the population will be in Hardy-Weinberg equilibrium, as is well known (see e.g. Mayo 2008 for review). Hardy–Weinberg equilibrium (HWE) is the state of the genotypic frequencies of two alleles of a single gene (locus) after one generation of random mating in this infinitely large population with discrete generations, in the absence of migration, mutation and selection: if the alleles are A_1 and A_2 with frequencies p and q (= 1-p), then the equilibrium gene frequencies are just p and q and the equilibrium genotypic frequencies for $A_1 A_1$, $A_1 A_2$ and $A_2 A_2$ are p^2, $2pq$ and q^2. Thus, there is equilibrium at both the allelic and the genotypic level. Table 1 gives the frequencies for the 3 genotypes revealed by gel electrophoresis of human red cell adenylate kinase in a number of European populations and one non-European population. (Here, q, the frequency of the rarer allele, is estimated as fr(AK_2 AK_2) + ½fr(AK_1AK_2).) This table illustrates differences among populations arising from geography and other factors, so that such variation can be used for purposes such as investigating the history of population growth, migration etc.

Population	Genotype			Sample size	Frequency of AK_2
	AK_1AK	AK_1AK_2	AK_2AK_2		
British	1720	165	2	1887	0.0448
Indian (England)	107	24	1	132	0.0985
Irish	739	50	0	789	0.0317
Finland	71	6	0	77	0.0390
Finnish Lapps	304	3	0	307	0.0049
Germany (Berlin)	1865	142	1	2008	0.0359
Germany (SW)	382	25	0	407	0.0307
Italy (Rome)	686	52	0	738	0.0352
Italy (Sardinia)	1004	28	1	1033	0.0145

Table 1. Genotype and gene frequencies for the red cell adenylate kinase locus in a number of samples from different human populations (extracted from Tills *et al.* 1971)

Most of the populations in Table 1 are in Hardy-Weinberg equilibrium, suggesting limited effects of disturbing factors, which include migration, inbreeding and natural selection. Now suppose that there is selection against all genotypes such that the fitnesses of the genotypes are as shown:

	$A_1 A_1$	$A_1 A_2$	$A_2 A_2$	Total
Fitness	α	β	γ	
Birth frequency	P^2	$2pq$	q^2	1
Freq. post-selection	$p^2\alpha/T$	$2pq\,\beta/T$	$q^2\,\gamma/T$	T

After selection, frequency (A_1) = p'

$$= (p^2\alpha + pq\,\beta)/T$$

The change in p,

$$\Delta p = p' - p$$

$$= (p^2\alpha + pq\,\beta - p\mathrm{T})/\mathrm{T}$$

If selection is not to alter gene frequencies, i.e. there is a gene frequency equilibrium, then $\Delta p = 0$ i.e. $p^2\alpha + pq\,\beta = p\mathrm{T}$, whence $p=0$ & $q=1$ or $p=1$ & $q=0$ or, non-trivially,

$$p = (\gamma-\beta)/(\alpha-\gamma-2\beta) \;\&\; q=(\alpha-\beta)/(\alpha-\gamma-2\beta)\,.$$

This last solution requires that $\alpha<\beta$ and $\gamma<\beta$. Hence, we usually write $\alpha = 1-s$ $\beta = 1$ $\gamma = 1-t$.

Related results hold for an X-linked gene and multiple alleles at an autosomal locus (see Mayo 1978 and Bürger 2000). The results for autosomal loci can be very complex: 'even in the absence of epistasis, mean fitness is not necessarily increasing; linkage disequilibrium may persist forever; and completely polymorphic stable equilibria may coexist.' (Bürger 2000, p. 51) (Here, epistasis is any interaction between non-allelic genes, not simply the suppression of the effect of one gene by another non-allelic gene.)

Following Fisher's pioneering work, Ford (1940, 1964) redefined genetic polymorphism as 'the occurrence together in the same locality of two or more discontinuous forms of a species in such proportions that the rarest of these cannot be maintained merely by recurrent mutation.' Ford then emphasised that such polymorphism could be balanced, as in Fisher's theoretical argument above, or transient, whereby neutral or nearly neutral alleles of a gene had frequencies fluctuating by chance, and all but one would eventually be lost from the population. Without this contrast, Ford could have been accused of assuming what he wanted to discover, namely, balancing natural selection, given that no alleles would be lost from an infinitely large population (and little was known of natural population sizes at the time), and that the rate of loss of genetic variability from large populations had been shown by Fisher and Wright to be very slow (Fisher 1922, 1930, Wright 1930).

Ford and others searched for balanced polymorphisms, and found some cases. An important one, which influenced much thinking over a long period (Mayo 2007), is sickle-cell anaemia in humans. Here, sickle-cell homozygotes ($Hb\beta^S\ Hb\beta^S$) have defective haemoglobin and can suffer from pernicious anaemia $\gamma=0.25$, heterozygotes ($Hb\beta^A\ Hb\beta^S$) are resistant to malaria and have normal erythrocytes $\beta=1$, and normal homozygotes suffer badly from malaria $\gamma=0.8$. This polymorphism results from one gene affecting two traits, rather than epistasis, two genes affecting one phenotype, though there are several other genes that affect response to the malaria parasite. Given the wastage through illness and death, there cannot be many such polymorphisms in a population at any one time.

Wastage (or suffering) is necessary to remove deleterious mutations from a population: as Sved (2007, p. 461) put it, "one 'genetic death' is necessary to remove a deleterious mutation, no matter how small the effect of that mutation.' These "genetic deaths", however manifested, constitute genetic load (see Morton 2007 for the history of the concept). If μ is the mutation rate to deleterious alleles at a locus, then the load is μ for recessive, 2μ for dominant mutations. One of the reasons for the idea of genetic load being discarded, except through acknowledgement of the 'burden felt in terms of death, sterility, illness, pain and frustration' as a result of deleterious mutation (Crow 1970) i.e. the human condition, as unfruitful has been the recognition of the sheer scale of variation at the DNA level, that is to say, polymorphism. For conclusive work on the theory of mutational load and how it relates to population variability, see Bürger and Hofbauer (1994) and Bürger (2000).

The concepts inherent in the stable equilibria discussed above are influenced by population size in three distinct ways. First, in a finite population there is a non-zero probability that one of the two alleles will be lost by chance. Secondly, in a population of effective size (the number of randomly mating individuals that give the same population dynamics as the population in question: Bürger 2000) N_e , with a mutation rate to new alleles μ for a given gene, 1+4 $N_e\mu$ alleles of that gene can be maintained (Kimura and Crow 1964). Equivalent results hold for X-linked loci (Mayo 1976, Nagylaki 1992). Thus, observation of polymorphism of a gene need have no implication in regard to selection. Thirdly, if $s>5t$ or $t>5s$ and $2N_e(s+t)<8$, the polymorphism will actually be lost rapidly from the population (Robertson 1962, Ewens and Thomson 1970). Mayo (1971, p. 329) noted that, 'although tetraploidy enhances the conservation of variation in small populations, it does not appear to do so by a factor of 2, as might have been expected from a doubling of the amount of genetic material.'

3. Linkage equilibrium

Suppose that there are two genes, A with alleles A_1, A_2 having frequencies p_A, q_A and B with alleles B_1, B_2 having frequencies p_B, q_B. There are 4 possible gametes

	$A_1 B_1$	$A_1 B_2$	$A_2 B_1$	$A_2 B_2$
frequencies	x_1	x_2	x_3	x_4
equilibrium	$p_A p_B$	$p_A p_B$	$q_A p_B$	$q_A q_B$

At equilibrium,

$$x_1 x_4 = x_2 x_3$$

The departure from equilibrium, $D = x_1x_4 - x_2x_3$ is termed 'linkage disequilibrium' (LD). It is easy to show (see e.g. Bürger 2000) that if the recombination between the A and B loci is c and LD in generation t is D, then in generation t+1 it is $D' = (1-c)D$. If the genes are unlinked, $D' = ½D$. If linkage is very tight, i.e. $c<<0.5$, D will decline very slowly.

The importance of observed values of D can readily be tested statistically, because on the hypothesis that $D = 0$, $nD^2/(p_A p_B\ q_A\ q_B)$ will be distributed approximately as χ^2 with one degree of freedom. (Because it is the square of the correlation between the loci, $r^2 = d^2 / p_A(1-p_A)\ p_B\ (1-p_B)$ is frequently used as the variable of interest.) For more than two alleles, equivalent results have been presented by Zaykin *et al.* (2008). Although much more complex because of the volume of data to be analysed, the analysis of LD data rests on modest, well understood statistical tools.

From the discussion above, LD between closely related polymorphisms is expected to be the norm, if there are large numbers of polymorphisms, unless these arose in linkage equilibrium and all populations are very large. Now several million single nucleotide polymorphisms (SNPs; section 5) are known within human populations, which means that the mean distance between human SNPs is about 1000 base pairs, the genome having about 3,000,000,000 base pairs (International Human Genome Sequencing Consortium, 2004). In the important experimental animal *Drosophila melanogaster*, with a much smaller genome (<200,000,000 base pairs), a population may contain up to one million SNPs (Burke *et al.* 2010). Hence, it is to be expected that there will be many closely linked polymorphisms. To make this statement more strongly, note that if the average human chromosome is about 2.5 Morgans long in recombination terms, and contains over 100,000 polymorphisms, there will be about 400 polymorphisms/1% recombination. Hence, linkage disequilibrium must be the norm, unless, as noted above, most polymorphisms arose in linkage equilibrium with each other. Even in this unlikely eventuality, for which there is no evidence, finite population size would generate linkage disequilibrium rapidly (Haldane 1940, Sved 1968).

Because of these stochastic effects on linked genetic variation, populations that are reproductively isolated from each other rapidly become genetically different, and this fact can be used to estimate time of divergence and other attributes on relatively simple assumptions. For example, Sved (2009) has shown that k small populations of effective size will develop r^2 equal to $1/[1+4N_e\, c(1+(k\text{-}1)\rho)]$, where $\rho = m/[c(k\text{-}1)+m]$, m being the rate of migration between adjacent populations. Applying this simple model to African and European HapMap (see 7.2 below) data, Sved (2009) obtained an estimate of time of divergence of less than 1000 generations, if there were relatively little migration subsequent to the original separation. This estimate is about one-third of current minimum estimates of divergence time, illustrating both how models can oversimplify complex situations and how much more is to be learnt about migration out of Africa.

Maynard Smith and Haigh (1974) first quantified the effect of selection of alleles of one gene on a linked gene. They showed that such selection would generate disequilibrium on a chromosome, the effect decaying with increasing distance from the gene under selection. This effect, termed 'hitchhiking', is important when selection is intense or rapid. As a selected allele increases in frequency in a population, or 'sweeps through' a population, adjacent genes show allele frequency changes, and even mildly deleterious alleles of neighbouring genes may rise in frequency. Overall, many changes will be wrought by a selective sweep, and their interpretation may not be straightforward. For example, Rose *et al.* (2011) showed that selection for organophosphorus insecticide resistance in the Australian sheep blowfly, *Lucilia cuprina*, changed allele frequency at the primary locus, α-esterase, whose alleles conferred resistance but also changed frequencies at many adjacent loci, including altering structural polymorphisms. This work supports the general concept that micro-evolution of this kind depends 'primarily on pre-existing intermediate-frequency genetic variants that are swept the remainder of the way to fixation' (Burke *et al.* 2010, p. 587). In fact, as Burke *et al.* further conclude, a so-called 'soft sweep' of this kind is unlikely to lead to fixation because of fluctuating selective forces and the likelihood that the selected alleles have pleiotropic effects that are not advantageous.

4. Sex determination and related polymorphisms

Inbreeding is generally deleterious. Self-fertilisation is the most extreme form of inbreeding. The requirement for two sexes in most multicellular organisms helps to ensure avoidance of selfing. In most animals, the two sexes are involved in the production of offspring. The human XY chromosome male XX chromosome female is one example of many; sex-determination can be by alleles of one gene, or by a number of different chromosomal differences.

In an indefinitely large population, the XX-XY system is stable and leads to equal frequencies of the two sexes (Fisher, 1930). In a small population, there is a low but non-zero possibility that an entire generation will be of one sex, so that the population dies out. Any given Y (or X) chromosome will eventually die out, and (because of the association of the Y chromosome with family name in some human populations) this possibility was first studied and branching processes used, in studies of the disappearance of family names (Watson and Galton 1875).

All sex-determining systems have advantages and disadvantages. The XX-XY system, for example, allows the sheltering of lethal alleles in the heteromorphic segment of the Y (Muller 1932), and hence the steady loss of function from the Y: 'the genes of the Y have gradually undergone inactivating and loss mutations, from the effects of which the organism has largely been protected, through the continual presence of an X having normal ... allelomorphs. In other words, the Y has paid the penalty always exacted by the protection of continual heterozygosis, and the consequent absence of natural selection. The largely inert Y... must retain enough genes to allow it to act as the homologue of the X in segregation, if it is to persist at all, and, if any dominant genes exist or arise in it, which are advantageous to the sex in which Y occurs exclusively, they may be retained by natural selection' (Muller 1932 pp. 133-4). Graves (2006), with the aid of a great deal of study involving DNA polymorphisms, has taken Muller's prescient conclusions and confirmed or elaborated them: 'Thus many factors feed into equations describing the rate of degradation of the Y chromosome, and these make it difficult to predict how near to extinction the human Y really is. I challenge population and evolutionary geneticists to derive a meaningful model with predictive power. Essentially, the stochastic nature of many of the Y-major rearrangements and deletions on the negative side and acquisition of new male-advantage genes on the positive means that it is at the mercy of chance events. It seems unlikely that the human Y has achieved a stable state. It would take substitution of function of only a few genes to render the human Y completely redundant and permit its complete loss' (Graves 2006, p. 911). Engelstädter (2008 p. 957) is among those who have accepted Graves's challenge, and has concluded that 'mutations on the X chromosome can considerably slow down the [random loss of those chromosomes bearing the fewest deleterious alleles]. On the other hand, a lower mutation rate in females [XX] than in males [XY], background selection, and the emergence of dosage compensation are expected to accelerate the process.'.

In flowering plants, where the basic form is hermaphrodite, selfing would be possible and likely if additional outbreeding mechanisms were not available. There are many of these; see Bateman (1952), Mayo (1983) and Leach and Mayo (2005) for discussion. I shall consider one system, gametophytically determined self-incompatibility (s.i.), to illustrate the special nature of the associated polymorphism.

In the single gene (locus) version of this system, there is one gene S, with alleles S_1, S_2, S_3, S_4... such that a female plant S_iS_j can be pollinated and fertilisation effected by a pollen grain S_k where $i \neq j$, $i \neq k$ and $j \neq k$. Thus, all plants are heterozygous and the minimum number of alleles for a population to persist is 3. There is strong selection for equal frequencies of the three possible genotypes S_1S_2, S_1S_3, S_2S_3 but in a population of finite size N there is a very low but non-zero probability ($<3(½)^N$) that only two genotypes will be represented in the offspring of any generation. Recognition of this fact led to the concept of the quasi-stable equilibrium (Ewens 1964) and a great deal of subsequent theory. If there are only 3 alleles and a new allele arises by mutation in a very large population, then it is at a substantial advantage and will rapidly increase in frequency to its equilibrium frequency of ¼. In most natural populations of plants possessing this outbreeding mechanism, very large numbers of alleles are present. If populations are large, these alleles will not be lost, but with moderate population sizes, high mutation rates are required to maintain the numbers of alleles observed.

Multilocus versions of this system are known, representable as $S_{ij}S_{ik}$, i = 1,2,3..., $j \neq k$ = 1,2,3..., whereby each allele of each gene behaves independently in pollen grain and style, so that pollination is possible unless all alleles in a pollen grain are represented in the style on which the pollen grain is lodged. Thus, the separate self-incompatibility genes in the multilocus system can behave as if they were not individually involved in a systematic disruption of panmixia; the only impossible genotypes are those homozygous for all self-incompatibility genes. Under such circumstances, fixation of one of the genes is highly likely unless all alleles have exactly the same selective value. Fixation at all but one of the loci brings the system back to that described above, which is highly resistant to fixation or disruption, except by other genes (or s-i alleles) which permit selfing, in which case fixation follows rapidly (Fisher 1941, Mayo and Leach 1987, Leach and Mayo 2005). Given these considerations, it is at first sight remarkable that many s.i. alleles are very old, in the sense that they appear to have appeared before the species that bear them (e. g. Richman 2000). Clark (1997, p. 7731) has noted that modelling of s.i. systems shows 'that the coalescence time of alleles [evolutionary time since divergence from some common ancestor]varies inversely with the rate of origination of novel functional alleles, and that for reasonable estimates of the rate of origination of new alleles, such extremely old polymorphisms are not unlikely'.

Sheltering of lethals is possible in the single locus system but much less likely in the multilocus systems (Leach *et al.* 1986). This is one small advantage the multilocus systems provide. It is of course entirely possible that quite different advantages accrue to multiple s.-i. loci, e.g. protein stability from duplication of active domains (Bhaskara and Srinivasan 2011); population-genetic modelling of such advantages awaits their demonstration at the cellular and organismal level.

It is difficult to explain how the more complex systems have evolved, just as with complex sex-determining systems. An initial advantage to a duplicated gene under strongly selective conditions (e.g. a population bottleneck) plus the regularity of Mendelian segregation in a subsequent expanded population might explain an individual case, but not the persistence of such systems in many very distantly related species.

5. Polymorphism at the DNA level

In the discussion so far, 'polymorphism' has simply referred to variants of a single Mendelian gene. These variants, however, may be anything from a change in just one DNA base in a sequence to a duplication of a whole structural gene or other lengthy sequence. Haemoglobin variants may, for example, arise from a single base change in one triplet codon. The *S* self-incompatibility locus alleles are much more complex variants. The human haptoglobin polymorphism has a number of alleles, of which one is a partial duplication of another (Smithies *et al.* 1962). Structural polymorphism of chromosomes has been shown to be very widespread (White 1973).

A restriction fragment length polymorphism (RFLP) is a polymorphism detected by DNA digestion with a so-called restriction enzyme. The polymorphism is a difference in the location of sites among two or more homologous DNA molecules (chromosomes) at which the restriction enzyme cuts the DNA molecule. Thus, the alleles differ in length (size) and can be distinguished by gel electrophoresis.

Repeated sequences, called tandem repeats or satellite DNA, are classified by size: satellites are highly repeated, with the unit of repetition a thousand base pairs or more, so that the overall satellite is of the order of millions of base pairs in length; minisatellites are less repeated shorter sequences, 10-100 base pairs repeated sufficiently frequently give an overall length of thousands of base pairs; and microsatellites, which are shorter numbers of repetitions of sequences shorter than 10 base pairs. Satellites are found on Y chromosomes and near centromeres and telomeres, while microsatellites and minisatellites occur in the euchromatin of most eukaryotes. Minisatellites were the basis of most forensic DNA and much agricultural application until the recognition of how many SNPs there are.

Single nucleotide polymorphism, usually diallelic, and identified directly through DNA sequencing, has become very important since technologies for rapid DNA sequencing have become first feasible and now widely available. Development continues at a rapid rate (Rothberg *et al.* 2011). SNPs can occur anywhere in the genome, whether the DNA encodes structural genes, regulatory elements that are not translated, or DNA that is not transcribed. Although SNPs are now a vital tool for many kinds of investigation, their manifold effects are only beginning to be understood. For example, synonymous changes in codons (i.e. those that do not lead to a change in the encoded-for amino acids) in SNPs have been implicated in several diseases (Sauna and Kimchi-Scarfati 2011).

Table 2 lists some of the different types of possible polymorphism. RNA different from transcribed DNA expectation (e.g. Li *et al.* 2011) has not been included because its phenotypic polymorphic outcomes are not clear.

DNA variation	Example of polymorphism
Whole chromosome	Sex determination
Whole chromosome inactivation	
Part of chromosome	Translocation, deletion, inversion, duplication
Whole gene	Translocation, deletion, inversion, duplication Protein polymorphism e. g. human haptoglobin
Whole gene inactivation	
Part of gene	Translocation, deletion, inversion, duplication
Part of sequence	
Restriction fragment length polymorphism (RFLP)	
Short tandem repeat (STR)	
Variable number tandem repeat (VNTR)/microsatellites & minisatellites	
Single nucleotide	

Table 2. DNA polymorphism

At every level of analysis from the chromosome down to the SNP, polymorphism can be used to investigate problems from the individual (e. g. risk prediction) to the population (e.g. the value and utility of ethnic group classification: Romualdi *et al.* 2002).

6. Polymorphism and quantitative variation

As already noted, the relationship between phenotype and polymorphism has been under investigation since the discovery of genetic polymorphism. Well characterised human polymorphisms such as the ABO blood groups have been shown to influence many quantitative traits, as well as being associated with disease as discussed in section 7 below. George and Elston (1987) provided a reliable method of analysis for use in small-scale human studies. Thus ABO influences serum cholesterol level (Mayo *et al.* 1969 and many subsequent studies) but the mechanism for this small effect is unknown. The same comment applies to the attraction for mosquitoes of some ABO phenotypes over others (Shirai *et al.* 2000).

Allen *et al.* (2010) have shown, through a meta-analysis and other studies of over 2,800,000 single nucleotide polymorphisms in over 180,000 individuals, that genetic variants in over 180 gene loci influence human height. There are no useful tools for modelling this kind of causation, other than the statistical methods built on the work of Fisher (1918), which cannot provide insight into physiological mechanisms.

In genetics applied to plant and animal improvement, useful methods can be developed which allow genetic improvement without a knowledge of physiological or molecular mechanism. Marker-assisted selection is the most important of these. The idea of using linkage disequilibrium for selection is not new. It was recognised early that detection of one or more markers associated with an increase in a desirable trait could allow selection for the trait using the markers. In this case, the markers would be associated with a chromosomal region influencing the trait of interest, such a region being called a quantitative trait locus (QTL). The method has, however, only become practicable with the discovery and mapping of thousands of DNA markers. Guimarães *et al.* (2007) give an account of the development of the field. For an example of industry application of marker-assisted selection, see Johnson and Graser (2010). They studied 12 commercial (GeneSTAR®) markers in populations from different breeds (temperate: Angus, Hereford, Murray Grey, Shorthorn; tropical: Santa Gertrudis, Belmont Red) and estimated effects associated with the markers 'that varied greatly across traits, suggesting large differences between the markers for their utility as selection tools in these populations' (p. 1917). If a QTL lies in a known gene in a known biochemical pathway, it can have a meaning other than its association with the trait of interest, but the utility of the association does not depend on such knowledge.

If markers have to be discovered, evaluated and applied for each trait, progress will be more certain than with traditional methods of animal breeding, but it will be costly and only slightly accelerated. Meuwissen *et al.* (2001) made a major advance in marker-assisted selection. Rather than simply search for individual markers of sufficient biological significance to be worth using in a breeding programme, they proposed a radically different approach using linkage disequilibrium between QTL and large numbers of markers across the genome without mapping the QTL. They introduced novel Bayesian statistical methods for estimating breeding value based on differing prior distributions of the effects of QTL and showed that high accuracy could be achieved. In 2001, cost-effective genotyping of very large numbers of markers was unavailable, but the tools used in the Human Genome project (section 7.2) radically reduced genotyping cost. SNP chips became available, so that Meuwissen *et al.*'s method, termed genomic selection, began to be implemented. Many dairy cattle breeders in advanced countries have adopted some of these new techniques. From

Meuwissen *et al.*'s work (and see also Goddard and Hayes 2007), genomic selection should almost double the rate of genetic improvement compared with traditional progeny testing. It has been claimed to be the most important advance in animal breeding since Henderson's (1953) Best Linear Unbiased Prediction. It will be applied to plant breeding.

7. Human examples

7.1 Association between polymorphism and disease

As cryptic human polymorphisms were identified, from the ABO blood groups in 1900 onwards, and at the same time many common diseases seen to 'run in families' were shown to have moderate to high heritability, it was natural that associations between phenotypes of a polymorphism and disease phenotypes would be sought. Discovery of such associations was expected to aid in the elucidation of the role of polymorphism in quantitative variation and might have been expected to allow risk prediction if very strong associations had been discovered. These analyses required the recognition that a disease state was a clinical definition related to a point on a scale of underlying liability (in the sense of Rendel 1967).

Detection of an association was relatively straightforward. Consider the 2 x 2 table:

		Polymorphic phenotype		
		A	not-A	Total
	Present	a	b	a+b
Disease state	Absent	c	d	c+d
	Total	a+c	b+d	n

Then the ratio (a/c)/(b/d) gives the relative risk of disease in A and not-A persons. Table 3 gives a small number of well-established relative risks for blood group O as against blood group A. As noted by Bodmer and Bonilla (2008), these findings, though robust, have not been useful.

Disease	Relative risk
Duodenal ulcer	1.90
Gastric ulcer	1.19
Cancer of breast	0.92
Cancer of colon & rectum	0.90
Pernicious anaemia	0.80
Atherosclerosis	0.69

Table 3. Significant relative risk differences between ABO blood group phenotypes O and A for several diseases (extracted from Mayo 1978)

Once the methods of analysis had been developed, they were applied widely. The following data from two schizophrenia studies are reproduced from Mayo (1978):

Disease status	Schizophrenic		Non-schizophrenic control	
Blood group phenotype	O	A	O	A
South Australia	31	46	534	409
Lancashire	31	31	334	243

These data suggest a combined relative risk of 0.63 for schizophrenia between persons of blood group O and those of blood group A. This finding has not been confirmed in subsequent studies. In a similar way, many claimed associations of schizophrenia with other polymorphisms have been unsupported in subsequent studies (e.g. neuregulin 1 promoter polymorphism rs6994992: Crowley *et al.* 2008; D2 dopamine receptor gene *Taq1* polymorphism: Behravan *et al.* 2008; *Nogo* CAA 3′ UTR insertion polymorphism: Gregório *et al.* 2005; Interleukin 10 gene promoter polymorphism: Jun *et al.* 2003; *NOTCH4* $(CTG)_n$ polymorphism: Imai *et al.* 2001). Wray and Visscher (2010) give the best established associations as part of a thoughtful discussion of all of the issues in unravelling the genetical component of schizophrenia causation.

In some cases, for schizophrenia and for many other disorders, 'candidate genes' were considered likely to influence clinical outcomes. Other cases (like the ABO example above) reflected capability rather than expectation (see Edwards *et al.* 2011 for a broad discussion of this issue in biomedical research).

Even when a real and probably meaningful association is found, its interpretation can be complex (Table 4). Here, association of two behaviour-linked traits with a polymorphism means that both sets of behaviour would be needed to determine anything to do with mechanism, even if the finding were robust.

Caffeine intake	*ADORA2A* genotype		Odds ratio
(mg/d)	*CC*	*CT TT*	(95% CI)
	(numbers of persons)		
	All subjects (P for trend < 0.001)		
<100	150	100	1.0
100–200	261	129	0.7 (0.5, 1.0)
>200–400	1062	446	0.6 (0.5, 0.8)
>400	426	161	0.6 (0.4, 0.8)
	Non-smokers (P for trend 0.03)		
<100	127	78	1.0
100-200	216	96	0.7 (0.5, 1.0)
>200-400	714	291	0.7 (0.5, 0.9)
>400	174	71	0.7 (0.4, 1.0)
	Smokers (P for trend < 0.001)		
<100	23	22	1.0
100-200	45	33	0.8 (0.4, 1.7)
>200-400	348	155	0.5 (0.2, 0.9)
>400	252	90	0.4 (0.1, 0.7)

Table 4. Odds ratio of having the adenosine A2A receptor (*ADORA2A*) 1083*TT* genotype for caffeine intake among non-smokers and current smokers (extracted from Cornelis *et al.* 2007)

Failed replication of original associations has also occurred with many other important diseases. Diabetes is an example, and here it is noteworthy that newer techniques, in one particular case consideration of microRNAs, a class of regulatory molecule with broad but not yet fully defined or explicated function, can show how influence on disease is mediated by products of DNA sequences other than structural genes (Trajkovski *et al.* 2011). Basic inflammatory mechanisms will be important in the underlying of disorders like diabetes that are closely related to inflammation (e.g. Liao *et al.* 2011), but this does not mean that associations will be found through 'candidate gene' polymorphisms.

New techniques for screening gene products rapidly increased the number of polymorphisms that could be investigated, making chance associations likely and increasing also the chance of finding real but meaningless associations brought about by linkage disequilibrium. These association studies are based on the idea that polymorphic alleles of a gene (or alleles of an unknown gene in strong LD with the test locus) can contribute to disease risk, i.e. there is a causal relationship. This contrasts with the rare variant hypothesis 'that a significant proportion of the inherited susceptibility to relatively common chronic diseases may be due to the summation of the effects of a series of low frequency dominantly and independently acting variants of a variety of different genes, each conferring a moderate but readily detectable increase in relative risk' (Bodmer and Bonilla, 2008, p. 696). As noted further by these authors (loc. cit., p. 208) 'A critical feature shared by common and rare variants is that they do not give rise to a familial concentration of cases.' Yet many common chronic diseases show strong familial concentration, so these contrasted hypotheses cannot tell the whole story. (See also Mayo and Leach 2006.)

7.2 Human Genome Project

The success of the Human Genome Project was partly based on competition to develop new, faster, cheaper ways of sequencing DNA, both in the automation of the chemical analysis and in the statistical analysis that allowed sequences for large regions to be aligned after assembly from multiple overlapping shorter DNA sequences. Progress has continued to be rapid, so that sequencing costs have declined to the point where almost anyone in an OECD country could imagine having her or his own genome sequenced. This has brought new concerns, sharpening ethical concerns about the use of genetic information (for example, whether one should offer genetic risk diagnosis for a disease with no treatment, such as Huntington's) but also raises all the old ones: how should probabilistic risk estimates be used, e.g. those based on polymorphic disease associations? What level of risk requires medical or other intervention? And so on. These problems do not relate solely to polymorphism, of course.

More directly related to polymorphism is the strategy of large scale analysis. As the number of polymorphisms became almost indefinitely large through the Human Genome Project, and assay costs tiny relative to the cost of collecting the human disease and control samples, or other groups to be investigated, methods based on small samples collected on a 'one-off' basis and individual polymorphisms had to be discarded in favour of methods based on the whole genome, such as the genome-wide association study (GWAS). The GWAS has now been used for a large range of traits and diseases, from baldness (Hillmer *et al.* 2008; and see Abbasi 2011 for an insight into one of the genes that may be relevant) and eye colour (Liu *et al.* 2010) to neuroticism (Wray *et al.* 2008) and measured intelligence (e.g. Butcher *et al.* 2008).

Handsaker *et al.* (2011) give a good account of some of the strategic issues in population studies, and Allen *et al.* (2010), cited above, and the GWAS references in the previous paragraph set out what is necessary to conduct and then to combine many big studies using millions of SNPs. These strategic concerns do not, of course, mean that all the requirements of a single study of a single polymorphism and a single disease, such as how inferences should be drawn from sample to population, must not still be met.

Table 5 lists some applications of polymorphism to genetic and other biological problems. It now seems clear that each individual carries some 2.5 million SNPs and substantial numbers of larger DNA polymorphisms. Post-HUGO international collaborations such as HapMap, set up to 'determine the common patterns of DNA sequence variation in the human genome and to make this information freely available in the public domain' (International HapMap Consortium 2003, p. 789), are beginning to assess this variability at higher levels of organisation.

Field	Application
Physiology	Gene and isozyme number
	Origin of cells and tissues
	Chromosome and gene inactivation
	Somatic cell hybridisation
Family studies	Linkage analysis
	Disease risk prediction
	Paternity testing
Population studies	Association of genes and diseases
	Genetic distance between groups
	Phylogeny
	Taxonomy
	Quantitative variation
	Pharmacogenetics/pharmacogenomics
	Sensory perception

Table 5. Application of polymorphism

8. Interaction

Interaction between a small number of factors, environmental or genetic, can readily be evaluated using standard statistical genetics. Table 4 is one example. Another is an association between a polymorphism of the fibrinogen β-chain gene and one influencing fibrinogen plasma concentration. Fibrinogen level is a risk factor for ischaemic heart disease (Woodward *et al.* 1998), yet the two polymorphisms, which are strongly associated, are not risk factors. Hence, the effect on heart disease must come about through mechanisms not yet elucidated (Vischetti *et al.*2002).

Current knowledge suggests that interaction will be the norm for any carefully investigated trait, the understanding of the interaction depending on the level of investigation, which will almost always employ polymorphism as a tool. For example, Luo *et al.* (2001) used RFLP in rice to investigate heterosis in grain yield and its components and the contribution of epistatic interaction to heterosis. They obtained over 250 inbred lines from their F10 generation and mapped RFLP across them, assuming epistasis to be solely a digenic phenomenon. Growing the crossed varieties at 2 locations, they were able to assess the consistency of their findings. They found 30 quantitative trait loci (QTL) in toto: 7, 15 and 8 for panicles/plant, grains/panicle and 1000-grain weight, respectively. Just 1 QTL was the same in both environments. Furthermore, only 8 of the 70 possible main effects associated were significant at the 0.1% level chosen by the authors. Taken together, these results imply very high levels of genotype × environment interaction., and the authors concluded that '[o]verdominant epistatic loci are the primary genetic basis of inbreeding depression and heterosis in rice'. Thus, RFLP had been used to derive a novel and important conclusion, which has been supported by other agricultural genetics studies, e.g. Barendse *et al.* (2007).

As noted above, the relationship between the determination of the heritable component of quantitative variation and polymorphism has not been fully elucidated. Insights will come from studies of regulatory DNA on a scale as yet barely envisaged (Frankel *et al.* 2011). Before then, however, new methods will be needed for dealing with multidimensional interaction on a scale never before attempted (Mayo, 2011).

9. Conclusions

The term 'polymorphism' is an old one which has survived many stages of reinterpretation and redefinition. Originally, it meant frequent or widespread but apparently meaningless variation in a population. Next, with the acceptance and development of the theory of Mendelian inheritance, it became a genetic concept, and with the coming of an understanding of stochastic forces in populations, genetic polymorphism was seen as something maintained by selection, or as transient while alleles were lost through chance variation. This was followed by the 'load' era, during which concerns were raised about the amount of deleterious mutation and the burden that this placed upon a population, even though the additive genetic variance in fitness, which is critical for the rate of change under natural selection (Fisher 1930), is proportional to the genetic load (Fraser and Mayo 1974). Indeed, in some formulations, load was seen as resulting from a population's deviation from an optimum genotype (Crow and Morton 1960). Now that we know that any individual human being may be polymorphic at more than a million SNP sites (loci) (e.g. Allen *et al.* 2010), with equivalent results for other outbreeding organisms, the idea of an optimum seems even more far-fetched.

The Human Genome project has revealed that humans have 'only' 20,000-30,000 structural genes, i.e. genes coding for proteins (International Human Genome Sequencing Consortium, 2004). However, much more of the DNA is translated, and its function is not yet understood, and it represents, at one level, many more 'genes', all interacting with the environment (e. g. Zhang *et al.* 2011). In addition, as noted above, the vast extent of DNA polymorphism, whereby even a SNP is a pair of segregating Mendelian alleles, means that polymorphism is the norm.

Looking back, it appears almost surprising that the effects of individual genes have been detectable and measurable so easily in so many cases. This has depended on the severity of deleterious mutations, on the visibility of many phenotypic variants, and on the keen eyes of medical practitioners and plant and animal domesticators and breeders. At a simple population genetic level, the analysis of Ewens and Thompson (1977) explains for fitness how an individual gene's effects are manifested. An important future task is to relate polymorphic genetic variation to phenotypic variation phenotypic variation, whether for human diseases, production traits in livestock and crops, or fitness and other attributes of natural populations. Equally important, but not discussed in this chapter, is how polymorphism relates to gene regulation.

10. Acknowledgement

I thank CSIRO for my research fellowship and Carolyn Leach for improvements to the manuscript.

11. References

Abbasi, A. A. 2011 Molecular evolution of HR, a gene that regulates the postnatal cycle of the hair follicle. *Scientific Reports* | 1 : 32 | DOI: 10.1038/srep00032. Accessed 13 July 2011.

Allen, H. Lango and over 290 other authors. 2010 Hundreds of variants clustered in genomic loci and biological pathways affect human height. *Nature* 467 832-838.

Barendse, W., Reverter, A., Bunch, R. J., Harrison, B. E., Barris, W. and Thomas, M. B. 2007 A validated whole-genome association study of efficient food conversion in cattle. *Genetics* 176 1893–1905.

Behravan, J., Hemayatkar, M., Toufani, H. and Abdollahian, E. 2008 Linkage and association of DRD2 gene *Taq*1 polymorphism with schizophrenia in an Iranian population. *Archives of Iranian Medicine* 11 252-256.

Bhaskara, R. M. and Srinivasan, N. 2011 Stability of domain structure in multidomain proteins. *Scientific Reports* 1:40 | DOI:10.1038 | socp0040 1-8 accessed 22 July 2011.

Bodmer, W. F. and Bonilla, C. 2008 Common and rare variants in multifactorial susceptibility to common diseases. *Nature Genetics* 40 695-701.

Bürger, R. 2000 *The Mathematical Theory of Selection, Recombination, and Mutation.* John Wiley & Sons, Chichester.

Bürger R., and Hofbauer, J. 1994 Mutation load and mutation-selection-balance in quantitative genetic traits. *Journal of Mathematical Biology* 32 193-218.

Burke, M. K., Dunham, J. P., Sharestani, P., Thornton, K. R., Rose, M. R. and Long, A. D. 2010 Genome-wide analysis of a long-term selection experiment with *Drosophila*. *Nature* 467 587-592.

Butcher, L. M., Davis, O. S. P., Craig, I. W. and Plomin, R. (2008) Genome-wide quantitative trait locus association scan of general cognitive ability using pooled DNA and 500K single nucleotide polymorphism microarrays. *Genes Brain Behavior* 2008 7 435–446.

Clark, A. G. 1997 Neutral behavior of shared polymorphism. *Proceedings of the National Academy of Science* 94 7730-7734.

Cornelis, M. C., El-Sohemy, A. and Campos, H. 2007 Genetic polymorphism of the adenosine A2A receptor is associated with habitual caffeine consumption. *American Journal of Clinical Nutrition* 86 240–244.

Crow, J. F. and Morton, N. E. 1960 The genetic load due to mother-child incompatibility. *American Naturalist* 94 413-419.

Crowley, J. J., Keefe, R. S., Perkins, D. O., Stroup, T. S., Lieberman , J. A. and Sullivan, P. F. 2008 The neuregulin 1 promoter polymorphism rs6994992 is not associated with chronic schizophrenia or neurocognition. *American Journal of Medical Genetics B Neuropsychiatric Genetics* 147B 1298-1300.

Edwards, A. M., Isserlin, R., Bader, G. D., Frye, S. V., Willson, T. M. and Yu, F. H. 2011 Too many roads not taken. *Nature* 470 163-165.

Engelstädter, J. 2008 Muller's ratchet and the degeneration of Y chromosomes: a simulation study. *Genetics* 180 957–967.

Ewens, W. J. 1964 On the problem of self-sterility alleles. *Genetics* 50 1433-1438.

Ewens, W. J. 2007 Fraser and the genetic load. Pp. 402-408 in *Fifty Years of Human Genetics a Festschrift and liber amicorum to celebrate the life and work of George Robert Fraser.* (O. Mayo & C. R. Leach eds) Wakefield Press, Adelaide.

Ewens, W. J. and Thomson, G. 1977 Properties of equilibria in multi-locus genetic systems. *Genetics* 87 807–819.

Fisher, R. A. 1918 The correlation between relatives on the supposition of Mendelian inheritance. *Transactions of the Royal Society of Edinburgh* 52 399-433.

Fisher, R. A. 1922 On the dominance ratio. *Proceedings of the Royal Society of Edinburgh* 42 321-341.

Fisher, R. A. 1930 *The Genetical Theory of Natural Selection.* Oxford University Press.

Fisher, R. A. 1941 Average excess and average effect of a gene substitution. *Annals of Eugenics* 11 53-63.

Ford, E.B. 1964 (4th edn 1975). *Ecological genetics*. Chapman and Hall, London.

Frankel, N., Erezyilmaz, D. F., McGregor, A. P., Wang, S., Payre, F. & Stern, D. L.1 2011 Morphological evolution caused by many subtle-effect substitutions in regulatory DNA. *Nature* 474, 598–603.

Fraser, G.R. and Mayo, O. 1974. Genetical load in man. *Humangenetik* 23: 83-110.

George, V. T. and Elston, R. C. 1987 Testing the association between polymorphic markers and quantitative traits in pedigrees. *Genetic Epidemiology* 4 193-201.

Goddard, M. E. and Hayes, B. J. 2007. Genomic selection. *Journal of Animal Breeding and Genetics* 124 323-30.

Graves, J.A.M. 2006. Sex chromosome dynamics and Y chromosome degeneration. *Cell* 12: 901-914.

Gregório, S.P., Murya, F. B., Ojopia, E. B., Sallet, P. C., Morenoc, D. H., Yacubiana, J., Tavaresa H., Santos, F. R., Gattaza, W. F. and Dias-Netoa, E. 2005. Nogo CAA 3VUTR Insertion polymorphism is not associated with schizophrenia nor with bipolar disorder. *Schizophrenia Research* 75 5– 9.

Guimarães, E. P., Ruane, J., Scherf, B. D., Sonnino, A. and Dargie, J. D. 2007. *Marker-assisted selection: Current status and future perspectives in crops, livestock, forestry and fish*. Food and Agriculture Organization of the United Nations, Rome. http://www.fao.org/docrep/010/a1120e/a1120e00.htm accessed 17 August 2011.

JBS Haldane, J. B. S. 1940 The mean and variance of χ^2, when used as a test of homogeneity, when expectations are small. *Biometrika* 31 346-355.

Handsaker, R. E., Korn, J. M., Nemesh, J. and McCarroll, S. A. 2011 Discovery and genotyping of genome structural polymorphism by sequencing on a population scale. *Nature Genetics* 43 269-278.

Henderson, C. R. 1953. Estimation of variance and covariance components. *Biometrics* 9 226–252.

Hillmer, A. M., Brockschmidt, F. F., Hanneken, S., Eigelshoven, S., Steffens, M., Flaquer, A., Herms, S., Becker, T., Kortüm, A.-K., Nyholt, D. R., Zhao, Z. Z., Montgomery, G. M., Martin, N. G., Mühleisen, T. W., Alblas, M. A., Moebus, S., Jöckel, K.-H.,,

Bröcker-Preuss, M., Erbel, R., Reinartz, R., Betz, R. C., Cichon, S., Propping, P., Baur, M. P., Wienker, T. F., Kruse, R. & Nöthen, M. M. 2008. Susceptibility variants for male-pattern baldness on chromosome 20p11. *Nature Genetics* 40 1279 - 1281.

Imai, K., Harada, S., Kawanishi Y, Tachikawa H, Okubo T. and Suzuki T 2001 The (CTG)n polymorphism in the NOTCH4 gene is not associated with schizophrenia in Japanese individuals. http://www.biomedcentral.com/content/backmatter/1471-244X-1-1-b1.pdf . Accessed 21 June 2011.

International HapMap Consortium 2003. The International HapMap Project. *Nature* 426, 789-796.

International Human Genome Sequencing Consortium. 2004 Finishing the euchromatic sequence of the human genome. *Nature* 431 931-945.

Johnston, D. J. and Graser, H.-U. 2010. Estimated gene frequencies of GeneSTAR markers and their size of effects on meat tenderness, marbling, and feed efficiency in temperate and tropical beef cattle breeds across a range of production systems. *Journal of Animal Science* 88 1917-1935

Jun, TY, Pae CU, Kim KS, Han H and Serretti A. 2003 Interleukin-10 gene promoter polymorphism is not associated with schizophrenia in the Korean population. *Psychiatry and Clinical Neuroscience* 57 153-159.

Leach, C. R. & Mayo, O. (2005) *Outbreeding mechanisms in flowering plants: an evolutionary perspective from Darwin onwards.* Stuttgart, J. Cramer (E. Schweizerbart'sche).

Leach, C.R., Mayo, O. and Morris, M.M., (1987). Linkage disequilibrium and gametophytyic self-incompatibility. *Theoretical and Applied Genetics* 73: 102-112.

Li, M., Wang, I. X., Li, Y., Bruzel, A., Richards, A. L., Toung, J. M. and Cheung, V. G. 2011 Widespread RNA and DNA sequence differences in the human transcriptome. *Sciencexpress* 10.1126science.1207018. Accessed 25 May 2011.

Liao X. , Sharma, N., Kapadia, F., Zhou, G., Lu, Y., Hong, H., Paruchuri, K., Mahabeleshwar, G. H., Dalmas ,E., Venteclef, N., Flask, C. A., Kim, J., Doreian, B. W., Lu, K. Q., Kaestner, K. H., Hamik, A., Clément, K. and Jain, M. K. Krüppel-like factor 4 regulates macrophage polarization. *Journal of Clinical Investigation,* 2011; DOI: 10.1172/JCI45444

Liu, F., Wollstein, A., Hysi, P. G., Ankra-Badu G. A., Spector, T. D., Park, D., Zhu, G., Larsson, M., Duffy, D. L., Montgomery, G. W., Mackey, D. A., Walsh, S., Lao, O., Hofman, A., Rivadeneira, F., Vingerling, J. R., Uitterlinden, A. G., Martin, N. G., Hammond, C. J., Kayser, M. 2010: Digital quantification of human eye color highlights genetic association of three new loci. *PLoS Genetics* 6(e1000934):1-15, accessed 20 July 2011.

Luo, L. J., Lia, Z.-K., Mei, H. W., Shu, Q. Y., Tabien, R., Zhong, D. B., Ying, C. S., Stansel, J. W., Khush, G. S., and Paterson, A. H. 2001 Overdominant epistatic loci are the primary genetic basis of inbreeding depression and heterosis in rice. II. Grain yield components. *Genetics 158* 1755-1771.

Maynard Smith, J. and Haigh, J. 1974. The hitch-hiking effect of a favourable gene. *Genetical Research* 23 23–35.

Mayo, O. 1971. Rates of change in gene frequency in tetrasomic organisms. *Genetica* 42 329-337.

Mayo, O. 1976. Neutral alleles at X-linked loci: a cautionary note. *Human Heredity* 26: 263-266.

Mayo, O. 1978. Polymorphism, selection and evolution, in *The Biochemical Genetics of Man* (2nd edition).

Mayo, O. 1983. *Natural Selection and Its Constraints*. Academic Press, London.

Mayo O. 2007. The rise and fall of the common disease-common variant (CD-CV) hypothesis: how the sickle cell disease paradigm led us all astray (or did it?) *Twin Research and Human Genetics* 10 793-804.

Mayo, O. 2011 Interaction between genotype and environment: a tale of two concepts. *Transactions of the Royal Society of South Australia* 135 113–123.

Mayo, O., Fraser, G. R. and Stamatoyannopoulos, G. 1969. Genetic influences on serum cholesterol in two Greek villages. *Human Heredity* 19 86-99.

Mayo, O. and Leach, C.R. (1987). Stability of self-incompatibility systems. *Theoretical and Applied Genetics* 74: 789-792.

Mayo O & CR Leach (2006) Are common, harmful, heritable mental disorders common relative to other such non-mental disorders, and does their frequency require a special explanation? *Behavioral and Brain Sciences* 29 415-416.

Meuwissen, T. H. E., Hayes, B. J. and M. E. Goddard, M. E. 2001. Prediction of total genetic value using genome-wide dense marker maps. *Genetics* 157 1819-1829.

Morton, N. E. 2007 Genetic loads half a century on. Pp. 431-435 in *Fifty Years of Human Genetics a Festschrift and liber amicorum to celebrate the life and work of George Robert Fraser.* (O. Mayo & C. R. Leach Eds) Wakefield Press, Adelaide.

Muller, H. J., 1914 A gene for the fourth chromosome of Drosophila. *Journal of Experimental Zoology* 17 326-328.

Muller, H. J. 1932 Some genetic aspects of sex. *American Naturalist* 66 118-138.

Muller, H. J. 1950 Our load of mutations. *American Journal of Human Genetics* 2 111-176.

Nagylaki, T. 1992 *Introduction to Theoretical Population Genetics*. Springer-Verlag, Berlin.

Rendel, J. M. 1967 *Canalisation and Gene Control*. London, Logos Press.

Richman, A. D. 2000 *S*-allele diversity of *Lycium andersonii*: implications for the evolution of *S*-allele age in the Solanaceae. *Annals of Botany,* 85 (Supplement A) 241-245.

Romualdi, C., Balding, D., Nasidze, I. S., Risch, G., Robichaux, M., Sherry, S. T., Stoneking, M., Batzer, M. A. and Barbujani, G. 2002. Patterns of human diversity, within and among continents, inferred from biallelic DNA polymorphisms. *Genome Research* 12: 602–612.

Rose, C. J., Chapman, J. R., Marshall, S. D. G., Lee, S. F., Batterham, P., Ross, H. A. and Newcomb, R. D. 2011 Selective sweeps at the organophosphorus insecticide resistance locus, *Rop-1,* have affected variation across and beyond the α-esterase gene cluster in the Australian sheep blowfly, *Lucilia cuprina*. *Molecular Biology and Evolution* 28 1835–1846.

Rothberg, J. M., Hinz, W., Rearick, T. M., Schultz, J., Mileski, W., Davey, M., Leamon, J. H., Johnson, K., Milgrew, M. J., Edwards, M., Hoon, J., Simons, J. F., Marran, D., Myers, J. W., Davidson, J. F., Branting, A., Nobile, J. R., Puc, B. P., Light, D., Clark, T. A.,

Huber, M., Branciforte, J. T., Stoner, I. B., Cawley, S. E., Lyons, M., Fu, Y., Homer, N., Sedova, M., Miao, X., Reed, B., Sabina, J., Feierstein, E., Schorn, M., Alanjary, M., Dimalanta, E., Dressman, D., Kasinskas, R., Sokolsky, T., Fidanza, J. A., Namsaraev, E., McKernan, K. J., Williams, A., Roth, G. T. & Bustillo, J. 2011 An integrated semiconductor device enabling non-optical genome sequencing. *Nature* 475 348-352.

Sauna, Z. E. and Kimchi-Sarfaty, C. 2011 Understanding the contribution of synonymous mutations to human disease. *Nature Reviews Genetics* 12 683-691.

Shirai, Y., Kamimura, K., Seki, T. and Morohashi, M. 2000. Proboscis amputation facilitates the study of mosquito (Diptera: Culicidae) attractants, repellents, and host preference. *Journal of Medical Entomology* 37 637-639.

Smithies, O., Connell, G. E. and Dixon, G. H. 1962 Chromosomal rearrangements and the evolution of haptoglobin genes. *Nature* 196 232-236.

Sved, J. A. 1968. The stability of linked systems of loci with a small population size. *Genetics* 59 543-563.

Sved, J. A. 2007 Deleterious mutations and the genetic load. Pp. 461-467 in *Fifty Years of Human Genetics a Festschrift and liber amicorum to celebrate the life and work of George Robert Fraser.* (O. Mayo & C. R. Leach Eds) Wakefield Press, Adelaide.

Tills, D., van den Branden, J. L., Clements, V. R. and Mourant, A. E. 1971 The world distribution of electrophoretic variants of the red cell enzyme adenylate kinase. *Human Heredity* 21 302-331.

Trajkovski, M., Hausser, J., Soutschek, J., Bhat, B., Akin, A., Zavolan, M., Heim, M. H., & Stoffel, M. 2011 MicroRNAs 103 and 107 regulate insulin sensitivity. *Nature* 474 649-654.

Vischetti, M., Zito, F., Donati, M. B., and Iacoviello, L. 2002 Analysis of gene-environment interaction in coronary heart disease: fibrinogen polymorphisms as an example. *Italian Heart Journal* 3 18-23.

Watson, H. W. and Galton, F. 1875. On the probability of the extinction of families. *Journal of the Anthropological Institute of Great Britain* 4, 138–144.

White, M. J. D. 1973 *The Chromosomes*. London, Chapman and Hall.

Woodward, M., Lowe, G. D. O., Rumley, A. and Tunstall-Pedoe, H. 1998 Fibrinogen as a risk factor for coronary heart disease and mortality in middle-aged men and women The Scottish Heart Health Study. *European Heart Journal* 19 55-62.

Wray, N. R., Middeldorp, C. M., Birley, A. J., Gordon, S. D., Sullivan, P. F., Visscher, P. M., Nyholt, D. R., Willemsen, G., de Geus, E. J. C., Slagboom, P. E., Montgomery, G. W., Martin N. G. and Boomsma, D. I. 2008 Genome-wide linkage analysis of multiple measures of neuroticism of 2 large cohorts from Australia and the Netherlands. *Archives of General Psychiatry* 65 649-658.

Wray, N. R. and Visscher, P. M. 2010. Narrowing the boundaries of the genetic architecture of schizophrenia. *Schizophrenia Bulletin* 36: 14-23.

Wright, S. G. 1930 Evolution in Mendelian populations. *Genetics* 16 97-159.

Zaykin, D. V., Pudovkin A. and Weir B. S. 2008. Correlation-based inference for linkage disequilibrium with multiple alleles. *Genetics* 180 533–545.

Zhang G., Chen, X., Chan L., Zhang M., Zhu, B., Wang, L., Zhu, X., Zhang, J., Zhou, B. and Wang, J. 2011 An SNP selection strategy identified IL-22 associating with susceptibility to tuberculosis in Chinese. Scientific reports |1:20| DOI: 10.1038/srep00020 accessed 29 June 2011.

Zhang, L., Hou1, D., Chen, X., Li, D., Zhu, L., Zhang, Y., Li, J., Bian, Z., Liang, X., Cai, X., Yin, Y., Wang, C., Zhang, T., Zhu, D., Zhang, D., Xu, J., Chen, Q., Ba, Y., Liu, J., Wang, Q., Chen, J., Wang, J., Wang, M., Zhang, Q., Zhang, J., Zen, K. and Zhang, C-Y. 2011 Exogenous plant MIR168a specifically targets mammalian LDLRAP1: evidence of cross-kingdom regulation by microRNA. *Cell Research* advance online publication 20 September 2011; doi:10.1038/cr.2011.158 accessed 26 September 2011.

6

Speciation in Brazilian Atlantic Forest Mosquitoes: A Mini-Review of the *Anopheles cruzii* Species Complex

Luísa D.P. Rona[1], Carlos J. Carvalho-Pinto[2] and Alexandre A. Peixoto[3]

[1]Universidade Federal do Rio de Janeiro / Polo de Xerém, Duque de Caxias - RJ,
[2]Departamento de Microbiologia e Parasitologia, CCB,
Universidade Federal de Santa Catarina, Florianópolis - SC,
[3]Laboratório de Biologia Molecular de Insetos,
Instituto Oswaldo Cruz, FIOCRUZ, Rio de Janeiro,
Brazil

1. Introduction

Anopheles (*Kerteszia*) *cruzii s.l.* (Diptera: Culicidae) has long been known as the primary vector of human and simian malaria parasites in southern and southeastern Brazil (Deane *et al.*, 1970; 1971; Rachou, 1958). Between 1930 and 1960, *An. cruzii* together with *Anopheles* (*Kerteszia*) *bellator* and *Anopheles* (*Kerteszia*) *homunculus* were considered the main vectors of malaria once endemic in southern Brazil. Vector control has reduced or even interrupted malaria transmission in some areas, but *An. cruzii* is still responsible for several oligosymptomatic malaria cases in southern and southeastern Brazil. This mosquito is also a vector of simian malaria in Rio de Janeiro and São Paulo States (Deane et al., 1970). Studies on seasonal and vertical distribution of *An. cruzii* demonstrated high vertical mobility from ground level to tree tops and this behavior could be responsible for human infection by simian *Plasmodium* species (Deane et al., 1984; Marrelli et al., 2007; Ueno et al., 2007).

The distribution of this mosquito follows the coast of the Brazilian Atlantic forest (Consoli & Lourenço-de-Oliveira, 1994; Zavortink, 1973), which provides an excellent environment for *An. cruzii*, since it is an ecosystem abundant in bromeliads, the larval habitat for this anopheline (Pittendrigh, 1949; Rachou, 1958; Veloso *et al.*, 1956). The adults are found in a variety of habitats, from sea level in coastal areas to the mountains. Females are strongly anthropophilic and blood-feed preferably during the evening (Aragão, 1964; Corrêa *et al.*, 1961; Veloso *et al.*, 1956), perhaps biting more than one host to complete egg maturation, which is epidemiologically relevant for malaria transmission (Bona & Navarro-Silva, 2006; Wilkerson & Peyton, 1991). However, notwithstanding its importance as a malaria vector, there are not many population genetic studies of *An. cruzii* (e.g. Calado *et al.*, 2006; Carvalho-Pinto & Lourenço-de-Oliveira, 2004; Malafronte *et al.*, 2007; Ramirez & Dessen, 2000a,b; see also below).

The possibility that *An. cruzii* could represent more than one species was first suggested by morphological differences observed among populations from the states of Santa Catarina and Rio de Janeiro (Zavortink, 1973). Later it was revealed that southern and southeastern Brazilian populations of *An. cruzii* are polymorphic for chromosomal inversions (Ramirez *et al.*, 1994; Ramirez & Dessen, 1994). The authors found evidence for the occurrence of genetically distinct *An. cruzii* populations with three different sets of inversions on the *X* chromosome, defined as forms A, B and C. In populations where two forms are sympatric no heterozygotes were detected, suggesting the absence or limited gene flow between the two groups (Ramirez *et al.*, 1994; Ramirez & Dessen, 1994, 2000a,b).

The possibility that *An. cruzii* may represent a complex of cryptic species was also supported by isoenzymatic profiles from 10 distinct *loci* of several *An. cruzii* populations. This analysis indicated two genetically isolated groups, one from northeastern Brazil (Itaparica Island - Bahia State) and the other from southeastern and southern Brazil (Nova Iguaçu - Rio de Janeiro State, Cananéia - São Paulo State and Florianópolis - Santa Catarina State) (Carvalho-Pinto & Lourenço-de-Oliveira, 2004).

These papers, which proposed that *An. cruzii* is a species complex, led to further studies using molecular markers to investigate the genetic differentiation among populations of this malaria vector. For example, Malafronte *et al* (2007) found some differences between ITS2 sequences comparing a number of southern and southeastern *An. cruzii* populations from Brazil. Similar results were observed by Calado *et al* (2006), using PCR-RAPD and PCR-RFLP of the ITS2 region.

We used a number of single-copy genes to investigate the molecular differentiation and gene flow among the putative sibling species of this complex (Rona *et al.*, 2009, 2010a,b). The results and the main conclusions of these analyses are discussed in more detail below.

2. Molecular markers and the genetic differentiation among Brazilian populations of *An. cruzii s.l.*

The *timeless* gene is a *locus* involved in the control of circadian activity rhythms in *Drosophila* (reviewed in Hardin 2005). It also controls mating rhythms (Sakai & Ishida, 2001) and its orthologues in mosquitoes are potentially involved in maintaining temporal reproductive isolation between closely related species. Rona *et al* (2009) isolated a fragment of the *timeless* gene in *An. cruzii* and used it to assess the genetic differentiation among six populations of this malaria vector within its geographic distribution range in Brazil: Florianópolis - Santa Catarina State, Cananéia and Juquitiba - São Paulo State, Itatiaia - Rio de Janeiro State, Santa Teresa - Espírito Santo State and Itaparica Island - Bahia State (Figure 1).

Very strong evidence was obtained for the existence of a different species in Itaparica, a finding that supports the isoenzyme study mentioned above (Carvalho-Pinto & Lourenço-de-Oliveira, 2004). Extremely high F_{ST} values and an elevated number of fixed differences (Table 1) were observed between this northeastern population and the other five studied localities. In addition, the data also suggest that some populations from southern and southeastern regions might also constitute different incipient species. Moderately high F_{ST} values were found when comparing Itatiaia with Florianópolis, Cananéia, Juquitiba and Santa Teresa, suggesting perhaps that this population is in a process of differentiation and incipient speciation (Table 1).

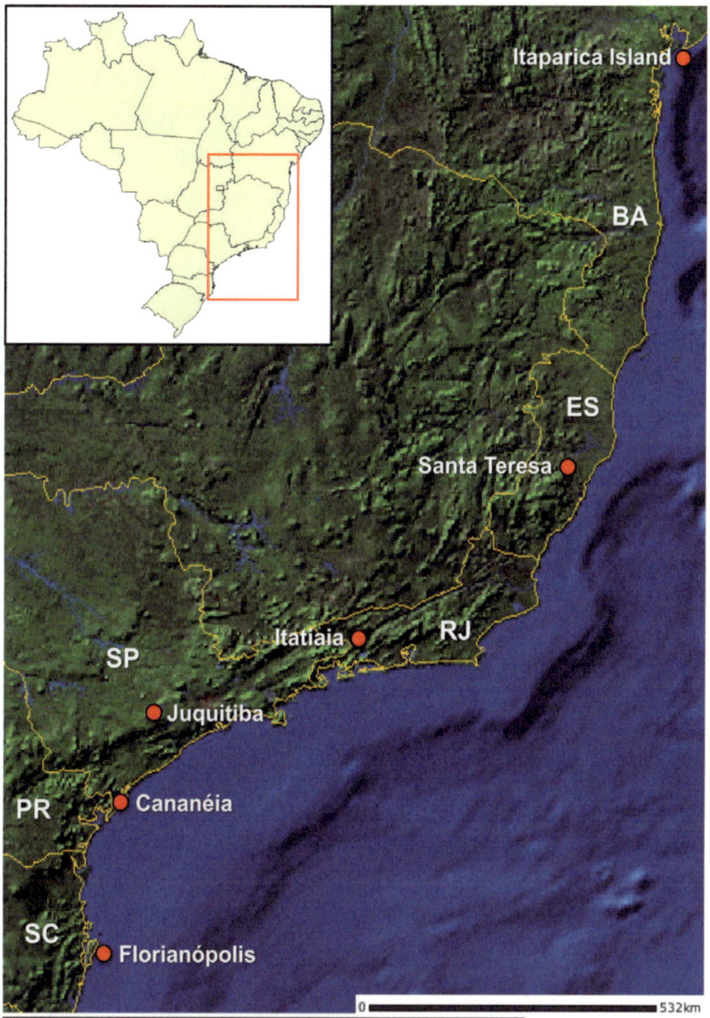

	Florianópolis	Cananéia	Juquitiba	Itatiaia	Santa Teresa
Cananéia	283	-			
Juquitiba	421	146	-		
Itatiaia	688	440	303	-	
Santa Teresa	1166	938	800	495	-
Itaparica	1890	1633	1485	1200	800

Fig. 1. Localities of the six Brazilian *An. cruzii* populations studied in Rona *et al.* (2009). Values in table are approximated distances between localities in km. (Source: IBGE and Google Maps). All mosquitoes used in this study were females captured at the following localities along the Brazilian Atlantic forest: Florianópolis, Santa Catarina State (SC) (27°31′S / 48°30′W), Cananéia and Juquitiba, São Paulo State (SP) (25°01′S / 47°55′W and 23°57′S / 47°03′W), Itatiaia, Rio de Janeiro State (RJ) (22°27′S / 44°36′W), Santa Teresa, Espírito Santo State (ES) (19°56′S / 40°35′W) and Itaparica Island (Jaguaripe), Bahia State (BA) (13°05′S / 38°48′W) (Modified from Rona *et al.*, 2009).

	Florianópolis	Cananéia	Juquitiba	Itatiaia	Santa Teresa	Itaparica (Bahia)
Florianópolis	-	0.055	0.087	0.145	0.158	0.835
Cananéia	00	-	0.108	0.225	0.215	0.851
Juquitiba	00	00	-	0.203	0.069	0.840
Itatiaia	00	00	00	-	0.184	0.876
Santa Teresa	00	00	00	00	-	0.862
Itaparica (Bahia)	27	29	30	30	32	-

Table 1. Genetic differentiation between *An. cruzii* populations using the *timeless* gene. The pair-wise estimates of population differentiation (F_{ST}) are shown in the upper right matrix and the numbers of fixed differences between each pair of populations are shown in the lower left matrix of the table. In all cases the F_{ST} values were significant (significance evaluated by 1000 random permutations). The sequences were aligned using ClustalX software (Thompson *et al.*, 1997) and population genetics analysis was carried out using DNASP4.0 (Rozas *et al.*, 2003) and ProSeq v 2.91 (Filatov & Charlesworth, 1999) (Modified from Rona *et al.*, 2009).

These results were supported by a Neighbor-joining tree (Figure 2). The *An. cruzii* sequences from Itaparica (Bahia) were clearly separated in an isolated branch indicating that this northeastern population has diverged significantly from the other populations, in agreement with the isoenzyme analysis (Carvalho-Pinto & Lourenço-de-Oliveira, 2004). In addition, although no clear separation between the *timeless* sequences from Florianópolis, Cananéia, Juquitiba and Santa Teresa was observed, the sequences from Itatiaia do not appear at a random, showing some clustering. Therefore, a process of incipient speciation seems to be occurring between Itatiatia and the other studied southern and southeastern populations.

To investigate in more detail the genetic differentiation between the southern/southeastern and northeastern siblings of *An. cruzii*, a *multilocus* analysis was carried out comparing Itaparica to Florianópolis (Rona *et al.*, 2010a). The aim of this study was to determine if there is still gene flow between the two sibling species and to estimate their divergence time. This analysis was implemented using six *loci*, three circadian clock genes (*timeless*, *Clock* and *cycle)* and three encoding ribosomal proteins (*Rp49*, *RpS29* and *RpS2)*. As mentioned above, circadian clock genes (Hardin, 2005), such as *timeless*, *Clock* and *cycle*, are putatively involved in the control of mating rhythms and therefore are potentially important in maintaining temporal reproductive isolation between closely related species (Sakai & Ishida, 2001, Tauber *et al.*, 2003). The analysis revealed very high F_{ST} values (ranging from 0.58 to 0.89) and fixed differences between these two cryptic species in all six *loci*, irrespective of their function. The divergence time and the migration rate parameters were estimated for all combined *loci*. Figure 3 shows the posterior probability distributions for each of the three parameters estimated using the IM program. The results suggested that the two species have not exchanged migrants since their separation and that they possibly diverged between 1.1 and 3.6 million years ago (Rona *et al.*, 2010a). In fact, the divergence time between the southern and northeastern species fall within the Pleistocene, a period of intense climatic changes (Cantolla, 2003; Ravelo *et al.*, 2004).

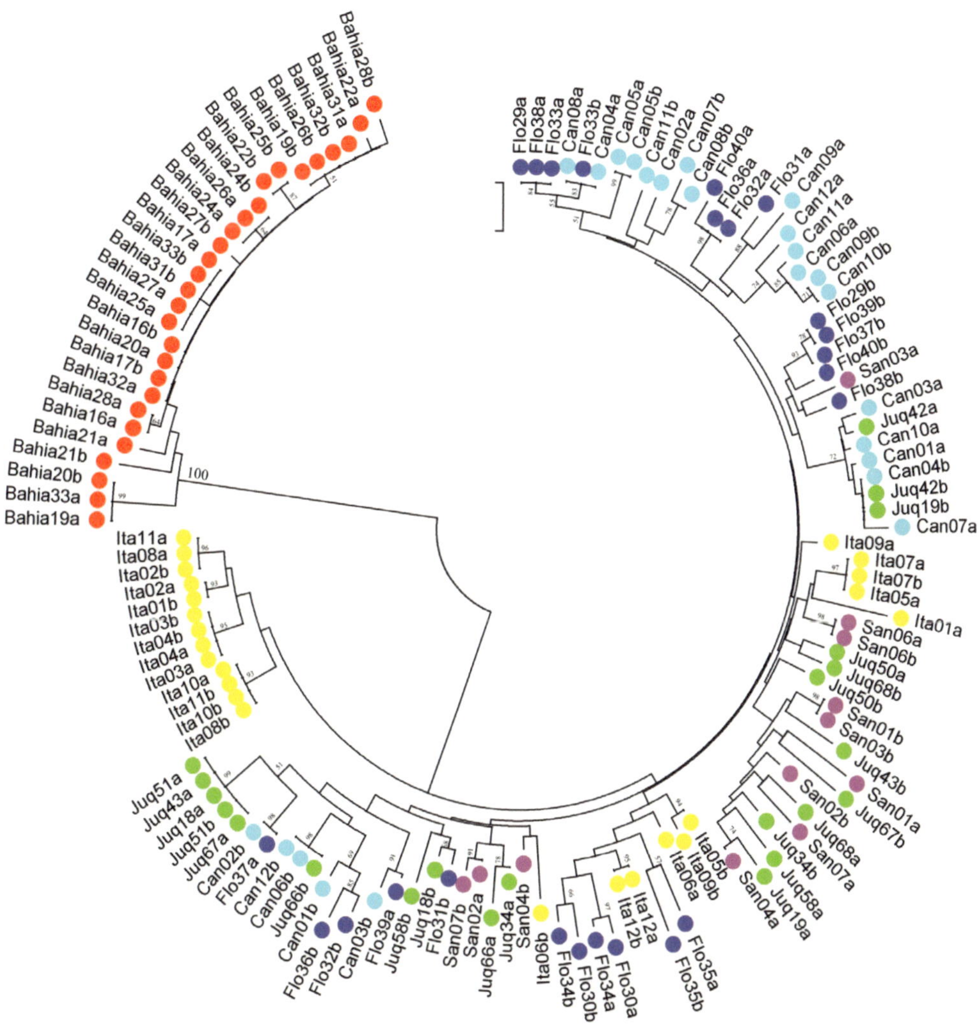

Fig. 2. Neighbor-joining tree using *timeless* nucleotide sequences of the *Anopheles cruzii* populations carried out using MEGA 4.0 (Tamura *et al.*, 2007) with Kimura 2-parameters distance. Numbers on the nodes represent the percentage bootstrap values based on 1000 replications. Flo: Florianópolis population; Can: Cananéia; Juq: Juquitiba; Ita: Itatiaia; San: Santa Teresa; Bahia: Itaparica Island population. (Source: Rona *et al.*, 2009).

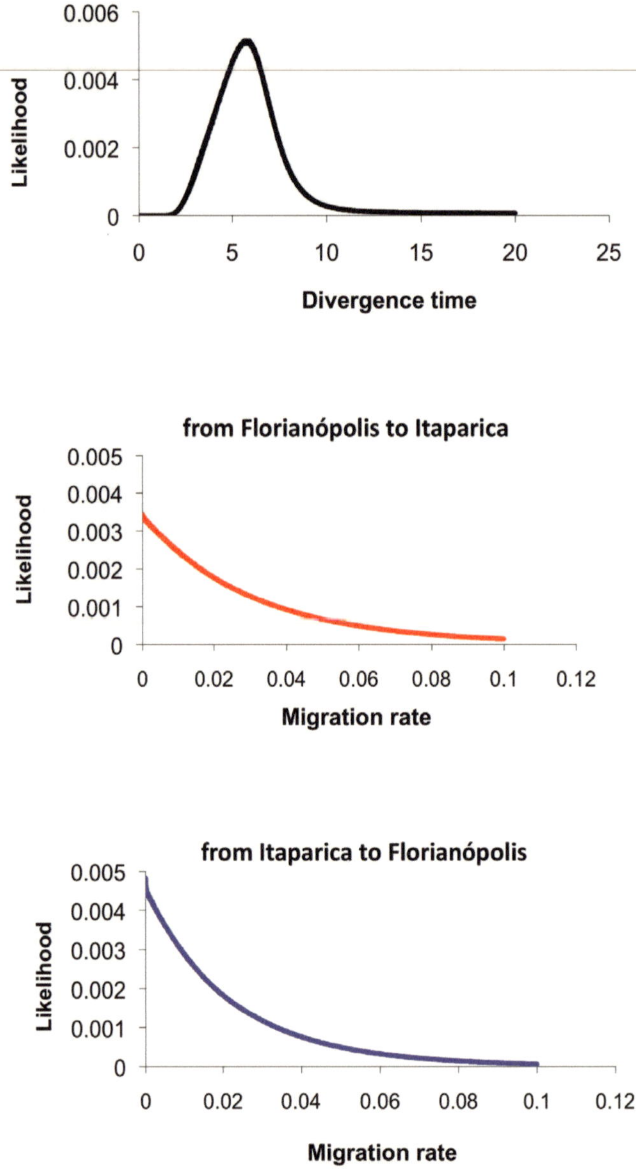

Fig. 3. Posterior probability distributions for each of the three demographic parameters estimated using IM: divergence time between Florianópolis and Itaparica, and migration rates in both directions. The estimated mutation rate, based on Drosophila, was used to convert the divergence time parameter *t* to the number of years since population splitting. Four IM simulations using different seed numbers were plotted for each parameter estimate. All curves are shown including the range of the priors. The IM program is an implementation of the Isolation with Migration model and is based on the MCMC (Markov Chain Monte Carlo) simulations of genealogies (Hey & Nielsen, 2004). Initial IM runs were performed in order to establish appropriate upper limits for the priors of each demographic parameter mentioned above. These preliminary simulations generated marginal

distributions that facilitated the choice of parameter values used in the final IM analyses. The convergence was assessed through multiple long runs (four independent MCMC runs with different seed numbers were carried out with at least 30,000,000 recorded steps after a burn-in of 100,000 steps) and by monitoring the ESS values, the update acceptance rates and the trend lines. The Infinite Sites model (Kimura, 1969) was chosen as the mutation model in the IM simulations because the two species are closely related and all genes are nuclear. The optimal recombination-filtered block was extracted from each gene alignment using the IM_{GC} program, which also removes haplotypes that represent likely recombinant sequences (Woerner *et al.*, 2007). See Rona *et al.* (2010a) for more details. (Modified from Rona *et al.*, 2010a).

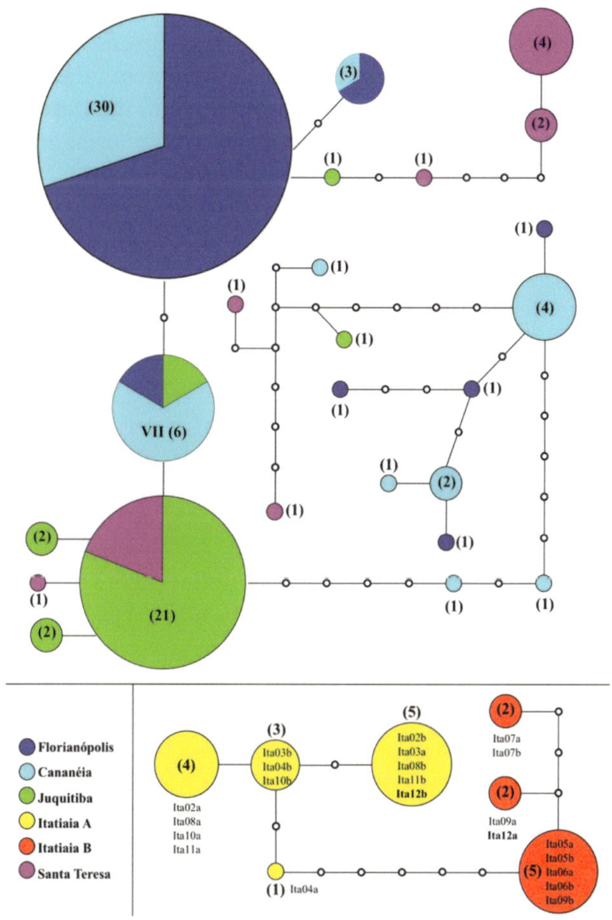

Fig. 4. Haplotype network of *cpr* sequences. Each color represents one population of *An. cruzii*. Each circle represents a different haplotype with size proportional to its relative frequency. The number of sequences of each haplotype is given in brackets. The small white circles represent missing intermediates and the lines connecting the haplotypes represent one mutational step between two observed haplotypes. Each individual of Itatiaia population is discriminated next to the respective haplotype. The haplotype network was estimated using TCS1.21 (Clement *et al.*, 2000). (Modified from Rona *et al.*, 2010b).

As mentioned above, the analysis of the molecular polymorphism and genetic differentiation of the *timeless* gene among *An. cruzii* populations from southern and southeastern Brazil suggested that the population from Itatiaia (Rio de Janeiro State) is in a process of differentiation and incipient speciation (Rona *et al.*, 2009). To analyze the divergence between these populations, a fragment of the *cpr* gene, a *locus* involved in metabolic insecticide resistance and odorant clearance in insects, was used. High F_{ST} values, some fixed differences and few shared polymorphisms were found between Itatiaia and the other populations (Florianópolis, Cananéia, Juquitiba and Santa Teresa). Moreover, an haplotype network constructed using the *cpr* sequences shows that Itatiaia is clearly separated in an isolated group (Figure 4) suggesting that this population represents a different species in the *An. cruzii* complex (Rona *et al.*, 2010b).

In addition, a more detailed analysis of the Itatiaia *cpr* sequences revealed that this sample might enclose two different sets of individuals. Based on the number of uninterrupted AG repeats found in the intron included in the studied fragment, the Itatiaia population can be divided in two groups: one called Itatiaia A (04 to 06 AG repeats) and the second, called Itatiaia B (03 AG repeats) (Figure 5). In fact, the separation between the two groups is also

Ita02a	AGAGAGAGAG
Ita02b	AGAGAGAGAGAG
Ita03a	AGAGAGAGAGAG
Ita03b	AGAGAGAGAG
Ita04a	AGAGAGAG
Ita04b	AGAGAGAGAG
Ita05a/b	AGAGAG
Ita06a/b	AGAGAG
Ita07a/b	AGAGAG
Ita08a	AGAGAGAGAG
Ita08b	AGAGAGAGAGAG
Ita09a/b	AGAGAG
Ita10a/b	AGAGAGAGAG
Ita11a	AGAGAGAGAG
Ita11b	AGAGAGAGAGAG
Ita12a	AGAGAG
Ita12b	AGAGAGAGAGAG

Fig. 5. Schematic representation of the AG repeat variable region in the DNA sequences of the *cpr* gene fragment from the Itatiaia population. The sequences of homozygote individuals were grouped and are represented as a/b. The haplotypes with exactly three AG repeats are in red. According to this classification the individuals Ita2, Ita3, Ita4, Ita8, Ita10 and Ita11 belong to Itatiaia A (genotype "4-6/4-6"), the mosquitoes Ita5, Ita6, Ita7 and Ita9 belong to Itatiaia B (genotype "3/3") and individual Ita12 is the only "hybrid" between the two groups (genotype "3/4-6"). Inspection of the data shows that the Itatiaia sample is not in Hardy-Weinberg equilibrium suggesting the possibility that two sympatric sibling species might exist in this locality. (Modified from Rona *et al.*, 2010b).

evident in the haplotype network of *cpr* sequences shown in Figure 4. Besides, the F_{ST} value (considering gaps as single mutations) between Itatiaia A and B is quite large (0.67) and highly significant (P<0.001) despite the small sample sizes. To confirm, with another *locus*, the hypothesis that the Itatiaia population might include two incipient sympatric sibling species, the *timeless* data (Rona *et al.*, 2009) from the same sample were reanalyzed. As for the *cpr* data, the *timeless* sequences were divided into Itatiaia A and Itatiaia B. The *timeless* gene also suggests that the sequences might belong to two different sibling species with a highly significant F_{ST} value (0.34; P<0.001) (Rona et al., 2010b).

Further work is clearly needed in this locality and an analysis of a number of other molecular markers might allow a more precise estimate of the differentiation and gene flow between the two putative Itatiaia siblings and between this and other localities in southern Brazil. It will be also important to extend our analyses to a number of other populations along the distribution area of *An. cruzii* as this might provide a more complete representation of the evolutionary history of this species complex. These studies are currently under way.

3. Conclusion

In this chapter we reviewed some of our results on *An. cruzii* with emphasis on how the molecular data is providing insights on the evolution of this complex of cryptic species, an example of speciation in Brazilian Atlantic Forest Mosquitoes. Our results and previously published data from other groups suggest that this complex is formed by a number of siblings or incipient species with different levels of genetic divergence and gene flow.

Population genetic studies using molecular markers often revealed complexes of cryptic sibling species in Anopheles mosquitoes with wide geographical distributions (Krzywinski & Besansky, 2003). This is the case of the *An. cruzii* complex, an excellent model for studying ecological vicariance and endemic regions in the Brazilian Atlantic Forest due to its broad geographic range, from southern to northeastern Brazil, and its dependence on forested areas as larval habitat. The appearance of ecological barriers caused by climatic changes as in glaciation periods is a possible explanation for the genetic structure found in this species complex. *An. cruzii* is a forest obligate mosquito and these cooling periods are known to cause forest fragmentation (Cantolla, 2003; Ravelo *et al.*, 2004), which probably affected the distribution of intraspecific lineages and might have split a single ancestral species into isolated groups.

The genetic pattern exhibited by the *An. cruzii* complex is compatible with a historical scenario of populations isolated during the Pleistocene ecological changes (Carnaval *et al.*, 2009). The subdivision of the Brazilian Atlantic Forest has been recognized as a cause of endemicity, for example, in bats (Martins *et al.*, 2009) and pit vipers (Grazziotin *et al.*, 2006) and climatic changes have been proposed to explain the differentiation among many forest-obligate species (Carnaval *et al.*, 2009; Marroig *et al.*, 2004; Pedro *et al.*, 2008).

Understanding the forces that shaped the Brazilian Atlantic Forest diversity is essential to explain the biodiversity of this important and endangered ecosystem and might help the conservation programs selecting the endemic areas that should be considered conservation priorities.

4. Acknowledgment

The authors would like to thank Dr Rosely Malafronte (Instituto de Medicina Tropical de São Paulo), Dr Monique Motta (FIOCRUZ - Rio de Janeiro) and Claudiney dos Santos (Unidade de Medicina Tropical - Universidade Federal do Espirito Santo) for providing most of the *An. cruzii* samples used in our work. The authors are also indebted to Dr André Pitaluga for helping prepare Figure 1. Our work is supported by grants from the Howard Hughes Medical Institute, FIOCRUZ, Faperj and CNPq.

5. References

Aragão, M.B. (1964). Geographic distribution and abundance of *Anopheles* species (*Kerteszia*) (Diptera, Culicidae). *Rev Bras Malariol Doencas Trop*. Vol.16, pp. 73-109.

Bona, A.C. & Navarro-Silva, M.A. (2006). *Anopheles cruzii* parity in dense rain forest in Southern Brazil. *Rev Saude Publica*. Vol.40, pp. 1118-1123.

Calado, D.C.; Navarro-Silva, M.A. & Sallum, M.A.M. (2006). PCR-RAPD and PCR-RFLP polymorphism detected in *Anopheles cruzii* (Diptera, Culicidae). *Rev Bras Entomol*. Vol.50, pp. 423-430.

Cantolla, A.U. (2003). *Earth's Climate History*. Servicio Central de Publicaciones del Gobierno Vasco; [http://homepage.mac.com/uriarte/historia.html]

Carnaval, A.C.; Hickerson, M.J.; Haddad, C.F.; Rodrigues, M.T. & Moritz, C. (2009). Stability predicts genetic diversity in the Brazilian Atlantic forest hotspot. *Science*. Vol.323, pp. 785-789.

Carvalho-Pinto, C.J. & Lourenço-de-Oliveira, R. (2004). Isoenzymatic analysis of four *Anopheles* (*Kerteszia*) *cruzii* (Diptera: Culicidae) populations of Brazil. *Mem Inst Oswaldo Cruz*. Vol.99, pp. 471-475.

Clement, M.; Posada, D. & Crandall, K.A. (2000). TCS: a computer program to estimate gene genealogies. *Mol Ecol*. Vol.9, pp. 1657-1659.

Consoli, R.A.G.B. & Lourenço-de-Oliveira, R. (1994). *Principais mosquitos de importância sanitária no Brasil*. Rio de Janeiro: Ed. Fiocruz.

Corrêa, R.R.; Forattini, O.P.; Guarita, O.F. & Rabello, E.X. (1961). Observations on the flight of *Anopheles* (*Kerteszia*) *cruzii* and of *A.* (*K.*) *bellator*, vectors of malaria (Diptera, Culicidae). *Arq Hig Saude Publica*. Vol.26, pp. 333-342.

Deane, L.M.; Ferreira-Neto, J.A.; Deane, S.P. & Silveira, I.P. (1970). *Anopheles (Kerteszia) cruzii*, a natural vector of the monkey malaria parasites, *Plasmodium simium* and *Plasmodium brasilianum*. *Trans R Soc Trop Med Hyg*. Vol.64, pp. 647.

Deane, L.M.; Deane, M.P.; Ferreira-Neto, J.A. & Almeida, F.B. (1971). On the transmission of simian malaria in Brazil. *Rev Inst Med Trop*. Vol.13, pp. 311-319.

Deane, L.M.; Ferreira-Neto, J.A. & Lima, M.M. (1984). The vertical dispersion of *Anopheles (Kerteszia) cruzii* in a forest in southern Brazil suggests that human cases of simian origin be expect. *Mem Inst Oswaldo Cruz*. Vol.79, pp. 461-463.

Filatov, D.A. & Charlesworth, D. (1999) DNA polimorphism, haplotype structure and balancing selection in the Leavenworthia PgiC locus. *Genetics*. Vol.153, pp. 1423-1434.

Grazziotin, F.G.; Monzel, M.; Echeverrigarauy, S. & Bonatto, S. (2006). Phylogeography of the *Bothrops jararaca* complex (Serpentes: Viperidae): past fragmentation and island colonization in the Brazilian Atlantic Forest. *Mol Ecol*. Vol.15, pp. 3969-82.

Hardin, P.E. (2005). The Circadian Timekeeping System of *Drosophila*. *Curr Biol*. Vol.15, pp. 714-722.

Hey, J. & Nielsen, R. (2004). Multilocus methods for estimating population sizes, migration rates and divergence time, with applications to the divergence of *Drosophila pseudoobscura* and *D. persimilis*. *Genetics*. Vol.167, pp. 747-760.

Kimura, M. (1969). The number of heterozygous nucleotide sites maintained in a finite population due to steady flux of mutations. *Genetics*. Vol.61, pp. 893-903.

Krzywinski, J. & Besansky, N.J. (2003).Molecular systematics of *Anopheles*: from subgenera to subpopulations. *Annu. Rev. Entomol*. Vol.48, pp. 111-39.

Malafronte, R.S.; Marrelli, M.T.; Ramirez, C.C.; Nassar, M.N. & Marinotti, O. (2007). Intraspecific variation of second internal transcribed spacer of nuclear ribosomal DNA among populations of *Anopheles (Kerteszia) cruzii* (Diptera: Culicidae). *J Med Entomol*. Vol.44, pp. 538-542.

Marrelli, M.T.; Malafronte, R.S.; Sallum, M.A. & Natal, D. (2007). *Kerteszia* subgenus of *Anopheles* associated with the Brazilian Atlantic rainforest: current knowledge and future challenges. *Malar J*. Vol.6, pp. 127-134.

Marroig, G.; Cropp, S.; Cheverud, J.M. (2004). Systematics and evolution of the *Jacchus* group of marmosets (*Platyrrhini*). *Am J Phys Anthropol*.. Vol.123, pp. 11-22.

Martins, F.M.; Templeton, A.R.; Pavan, A.C.O.; Kohlbach, B.C. & Morgante, J.S. (2009). Phylogeography of the common vampire bat (*Desmodus rotundus*): Marked population structure, Neotropical Pleistocene vicariance and incongruence between nuclear and mtDNA markers. *BMC Evol Biol*. Vol.9, pp. 294.

Nei, M. & Kumar, S. (2000). *Molecular Evolution and Phylogenetics*. New York: Oxford University Press.

Pedro, P.M.; Sallum, M.A. & Butlin, R.K. (2008). Forest-obligate *Sabethes* mosquitoes suggest palaeoecological perturbations. *Heredity*. Vol.101, pp. 186-195.

Pittendrigh, C.S. (1949). The ectopic specialization of *Anopheles homunculus*, and its relation to competition with *An. bellator*. *Evolution*. Vol.4, pp. 64-78.

Rachou, R.G. (1958). Anofelinos do Brasil: Comportamento das espécies vetoras de malária. *Rev Bras Malariol Doencas Trop*. Vol.10, pp. 145-181.

Ramirez, C.C. & Dessem, E.M. (1994). Cytogenetics analysis of a natural population of *Anopheles cruzii*. *Rev Bras Genet*. Vol.17, pp. 41-46.

Ramirez, C.C.; Dessem, E.M. & Otto, P.A. (1994). Inversion polymorphism in a natural population of *Anopheles cruzii*. *Caryologia*. Vol.47, pp. 121-130.

Ramirez, C.C. & Dessen, E.M. (2000a). Chromosomal evidence for sibling species of the malaria vector *Anopheles cruzii*. *Genome*. Vol.43, pp. 143-151.

Ramirez, C.C. & Dessen, E.M. (2000b). Chromosome differentiated populations of *Anopheles cruzii*: evidence for a third sibling species. *Genetica*. Vol.108, pp. 73-80.

Ravelo, A.C.; Andreasen, D.H.; Lyle, M.; Olivarez, A. & Wara, M.W. (2004). Regional climate shifts caused by gradual global cooling in the Pliocene epoch. *Nature*. Vol.429, pp. 263-267.

Rona, L.D.; Carvalho-Pinto, C.J.; Gentile, C.; Grisard, E.C. & Peixoto, A.A. (2009). Assessing the molecular divergence between *Anopheles* (*Kerteszia*) *cruzii* populations from Brazil using the *timeless* gene: Further evidence of a species complex. *Malar J*. Vol.8, pp. 60.

Rona, L.D.; Carvalho-Pinto, C.J.; Mazzoni, C.J. & Peixoto, A.A. (2010a). Estimation of divergence time between two sibling species of the *Anopheles (Kerteszia) cruzii* complex using a multilocus approach. *BMC Evolutionary Biology*. Vol.10, pp. 91.

Rona, L.D.; Carvalho-Pinto, C.J.; Peixoto, A.A. (2010b). Molecular evidence for the occurrence of a new sibling species within the *Anopheles (Kerteszia) cruzii* complex in south-east Brazil. *Malaria Journal*. Vol.9, pp. 33.

Rozas, J.; Sánchez-DelBarrio, J.C.; Messeguer, X. & Rozas, R. (2003). DnaSP, DNA polymorphism analyses by the coalescent and other methods. *Bioinformatics*. Vol.19, pp. 2496-2497.

Sakai, T. & Ishida, N. (2001). Circadian rhythms of female mating activity governed by clock genes in *Drosophila*. *Proc Natl Acad Sci*. Vol.98, pp. 9221-9225.

Tamura, K.; Dudley, J.; Nei, M. & Kumar, S. (2007). MEGA4: Molecular Evolutionary Genetics Analysis (MEGA) software version 4.0. *Mol Biol Evol*. Vol.24, pp. 1596-1599.

Tauber, E.; Roe, H.; Costa, R.; Hennessy, J.M. & Kyriacou, C.P. (2003). Temporal mating isolation driven by a behavioral gene in *Drosophila*. *Curr Biol*. Vol.13, pp. 140-145.

Thompson, J.D.; Gibson, T.J.; Plewniak, F.; Jeanmougin, F. & Higgins, D.G. (1997). The CLUSTAL_X windows interface: flexible strategies for multiple sequence alignment aided by quality analysis tools. *Nucleic Acids Res*. Vol.25, pp. 4876-4882.

Ueno, H.M.; Forattini, O.P. & Kakitani, I. (2007). Vertical and seasonal distribution of *Anopheles (Kerteszia)* in Ilha Comprida, Southeastern Brazil. *Rev Saude Publica*. Vol.41, pp. 269-275.

Veloso, H.P.; De Moura, J.V. & Klein, R.M. (1956). Ecological limitation of *Anopheles* of the Subgenus *Kerteszia* in the coastal region of Southern Brazil. *Mem Inst Oswaldo Cruz*. Vol.54, pp. 517-548.

Wilkerson, R.C. & Peyton, E.L. (1991). The Brazilian malaria vector *Anopheles (Kerteszia) cruzii*: Life stages and biology (Diptera: Culicidae). *Mosq System*. Vol.23, pp. 110-122.

Woerner, A.E.; Cox, M.P. & Hammer, M.F. (2007). Recombination-filtered genomic datasets by information maximization. *Bioinformatics*. Vol.23, pp. 1851-1853.

Zavortink, T.J. (1973). A review of the subgenus *Kerteszia* of *Anopheles*. *Cont Am Entomol Inst*. Vol.9, pp. 1-54.

7

The Next Step in Understanding Population Dynamics: Comprehensive Numerical Simulation

John C. Sanford[1] and Chase W. Nelson[2]
[1]Department of Horticulture, NYSAES, Cornell University, Geneva, NY,
[2]Rainbow Technologies, Inc., Waterloo, NY,
USA

1. Introduction

Natural populations are always changing. Hardy-Weinberg assumptions are almost never realized because populations are seldom in equilibrium, and many random events (e.g., mutations, population size fluctuations, and environmental perturbations) irrevocably alter the genetic makeup of populations. Such genetic change can be either for the better (some populations adapt and expand) or for the worse (some populations shrink and become extinct). Change that occurs as the result of natural selection is termed *adaptive evolution* because natural selection favors the survival of organisms that are best adapted to their environments (i.e., have high fitness). On the other hand, *nonadaptive evolution* refers to change that occurs as the result of factors that act independently of organismal fitness (e.g., random genetic drift or mutation pressure). Because change within a population depends on so many variables and involves innumerable chance events, the study of population dynamics is both challenging and fascinating.

Geneticists study population-level change in three very different ways. The first approach is the empirical one. This involves the actual observation of living populations over time, and involves direct experimentation with the variables that affect population dynamics. One author (JCS) engaged in this approach the first 20 years of his career, first as a plant geneticist and breeder, and later as someone who was actively involved in plant genetic engineering. The empirical approach has the limitation that it is only possible to study changes that happen in a short amount of time, and which display effects that are highly visible or easily tracked. For example, when selecting for increased crop yield in plant breeding, it is only possible to reliably determine very substantial yield differences (roughly 10% or more) between genotypes, even with carefully replicated field trials. Such observations are very useful, but obviously miss most of what is happening at the genetic level (i.e., the innumerable subtle genetic changes that are happening within the population). While this empirical method has serious limitations, it has played a major role in the development of modern agriculture and modern medicine.

The second method is the historical/comparative approach. This involves observing differences (especially amino acid and DNA sequence differences) within existing populations and trying to infer population histories (e.g., see Li & Durbin, 2011). Such inferences can include the degree of relatedness between populations, the time of their divergence, and what parts of their genomes were affected by either positive selection, negative selection, or no selection. This historical approach is inherently limited by its various underlying assumptions, such as the concept of constant-rate molecular clocks or the neutrality of synonymous mutations. Because many exceptions to each assumption exist (e.g., see Sauna & Kimchi-Sarfaty et al., 2011 on synonymous mutations), the reliability and relevance of the historical approach has been hotly debated (for example, see Wilson & Cann, 1992 and Thorne & Wolpoff, 1992 on the molecular clock), but there is no doubt that it can sometimes help us to correctly infer certain genetic events in the past. There are a variety of computational tools that are designed to facilitate this historical approach in population genetics. These tools fall under the umbrella of bioinformatics, and include software packages that align sequences, infer phylogenetic trees, and perform various statistical analyses with the given data.

The third method is the theoretical approach. This involves studying how hypothetical or idealized populations might behave in forward-time, starting from a specific state, based upon our knowledge of genetics and population biology. Ten years ago one author (JCS) shifted his research focus from the empirical approach to the theoretical approach, because the theoretical approach allows consideration of the bigger picture and bigger questions.

The field of theoretical genetics was established primarily by mathematicians (e.g., Fisher, Haldane, and Wright). These scientists realized that even though mutations arise and segregate randomly, and survival is influenced by many random elements, and mating is largely random, still, directional processes such as selection can play an important role in shaping the genetic makeup of a population over long periods of time.

The mathematical approach to population dynamics has been very fruitful in terms of understanding numerous specific aspects of population change, when each is considered in isolation. This is particularly true, for example, where selection for a single trait is mathematically modeled, or where numerous neutral mutations are drifting in a population. The main limitation of the mathematical modeling approach is that it invariably requires extreme simplification of the model (e.g., just considering one or a few loci or mutations, or just one or a few variables). Unfortunately, real biological populations are not at all simple, and so there arises the possibility that the results of simplified mathematical models may not correspond to biological reality. This is especially a concern where theoretical models have become highly abstract, such that common sense can no longer help us gauge whether or not theoretical predictions are reasonable.

For these reasons mathematical models need to be tested. One way to do this is by returning to the empirical approach: studying living biological populations through many generations to validate theory. However, this is usually not practical, especially for organisms with long generation times. As a practical alternative, mathematical models can be tested in virtual populations using numerical simulation. It was for this reason that simple numerical computer simulations were first developed by population geneticists - to test and validate specific mathematical models.

Numerical simulations can be seen as the empirical enactment of real processes, but in a virtual environment. Even though numerical simulation experiments happen in a computer environment, numerical simulators can be used to conduct real experiments, and can illuminate processes happening in the real world. In terms of modeling fitness change over time, a good numerical simulation can act very much like an accountant's spreadsheet. Spreadsheets can be made to accurately and honestly reflect the true financial status of a corporate entity. Every dollar is tracked from beginning to end, as it comes and as it goes. In fact, in a large corporate entity, a spreadsheet is the only reliable way to see the big financial picture. Corporations and governments may not be able to trust their accountants, but they can at least trust the operation of their spreadsheets. Likewise, when numerical simulators are carefully designed to reflect the real world, they can be powerful and trustworthy tools. When used properly, numerical simulations can inform us about what is likely to be happening in the real world, even when direct observation is not feasible.

Population geneticists first used simple numerical simulation to validate a particluar component of genetic systems. However, as computational power has grown, and as the science of numerical simulation has become more sophisticated, we have now reached the point where we can analyze population dynamics in a comprehensive, integrated and empirical manner within a virtual environment, independent of copious and often very abstract mathematical modeling. Such simulation should enable us to obtain a more biologically integrated picture of how real populations change.

Seven years ago one author (JCS) had the opportunity to oversee the development of a comprehensive numerical simulator for the aforementioned purposes. Since that time, a group of biologists and computer scientists have been collaborating to develop a numerical simulator that can simultaneously model all the major known factors that affect genetic change, as well as their relevant interactions, to better approximate what occurs in the real world. The resulting program, Mendel's Accountant (Mendel), appears to be the first program that has seriously endeavored to do this. Mendel has been described in previous publications (Sanford et al., 2007a, 2007b), and is now beginning to be used for both research and teaching. This tool should not be viewed as a replacement for previous tools already developed within this field, but it is clear that it represents a major step forward.

2. Mendel's Accountant

Mendel's Accountant simulates genetic change within a population as it moves forward through time. Mendel does this by establishing a virtual population of individuals, and then precisely simulates mutation, selection, and gene transmission through many generations, always in the most biologically realistic manner possible. Mendel is unique in that it attempts to treat all aspects of population dynamics simultaneously and comprehensively, thereby ushering in for the first time the prospect of simulating reasonable approximations of biological reality.

Mendel's Accountant is an apt name for this program because it is largely a "genetic accounting" program. Every generation, huge numbers of specific mutations are introduced into a population, spread over the genomes of many individuals. Through the ensuing generations, some of these mutations are lost, while others increase in frequency. Each mutation must be tracked through many individuals and through many generations, along with all data that apply to that mutation (each has an allelic ID, mutational fitness effect, degree of dominance, and chromosomal location). During a large run, Mendel can track hundreds of millions of different mutations. Not only does Mendel do the genetic accounting associated with tracking individual mutations, it simultaneously does the genetic accounting associated with tracking: 1) linkage blocks as they recombine; 2) net fitnesses of each individual; 3) the distribution of the fitness effects of all the accumulating mutations; and 4) the resulting distribution of allele frequencies.

Genetic accounting via numerical simulation is possible because the underlying processes (Mendelian inheritance, random mutations, differential reproduction) are all relatively simple and mechanistic in nature and are therefore subject to straightforward accounting procedures. Furthermore, all the relevant biological variables are easily specified as parameters for use in simulation (e.g., population size, mutation rate, distribution of mutational fitness effects, heritability, and amount of selective elimination each generation). Like many high-performance numerical simulations, the core of the Mendel program is written in Fortran 90, allowing the execution of tasks that are extremely demanding computationally, making it possible to process huge amounts of genetic data.

To explain how Mendel works in the simplest way possible, it is useful to consider the series of decisions that an experimenter must make. Firstly, the experimenter must define the species and its reproductive structure. Is it haploid or diploid? How big is the genome, and what fraction is funcional? Is its reproduction sexual or clonal? Does the species ever self-fertilize? All these biological factors can be modeled by Mendel, and must be specified by the user, because they have a substantial impact on population dynamics. These parameters determine how reproduction and gene transmission will occur within the virtual species.

Secondly, the experimenter must define the characteristics of a particular population within the species. How big is the population before and after selection? Are there sub-populations? How many generations do we wish to observe? These parameters define the actual scope and architecture of a particular experiment.

Thirdly, the user must specify reproductive details. The reproductive rate must always be high enough to create a population surplus each generation, such that this surplus can then be selectively removed each generation. For example, the default reproduction rate is 3. In this case the number of offspring generated each generation is always 3 times larger than the specified population size. This creates a surplus population large enough for selection to remove two of every three offspring in the next generation. If the population under study reproduces sexually, recombination will occur at this stage. The experimenter must specify the number of chromosomes (assuming two cross-overs per chromosome) and the number of linkage blocks (this affects segregation of linkage blocks during gamete production).

Fourthly, the experimenter needs to specify the mutations that will be added to the population. After creating a new virtual population of offspring, Mendel then begins to add new mutations to those individual offspring. Mendel assigns mutations to individuals randomly, following a Poisson distribution. The experimenter specifies a mutation rate appropriate for the species under study (or one that is of theoretical interest). Likewise, the experimenter must specify a distribution of mutational fitness effects. Typically this distribution will include deleterious, neutral, and beneficial mutations. The mutations that are added to the population are drawn randomly from a user-specified pool of potential mutations (usually having a Weibull distribution of fitness effects). Drawing from such a distribution, some mutations will have large effects, but most will have small (nearly-neutral) effects (Kimura, 1983), as occurs in nature (Eyre-Walker & Keightley, 2007). Each new mutation has an identifier for tracking purposes, a fitness effect, a specified degree of dominance, and a chromosomal location (i.e., a designated linkage block).

Lastly, the experimenter needs to specify the nature of the selection process. Once Mendel has created a newly mutated population of offspring, it must implement selective removal. To do this Mendel first calculates the combined effect of all mutations in each individual (initial individuals containing zero mutations having a fitness of one, with beneficial mutations increasing fitness and deleterious mutations reducing fitness). Mutations can be combined either additively or multiplicatively (or in alternative ways, i.e., epistatically). Once the fitness of each individual has been calculated, a certain fraction of the population is selectively eliminated based upon genetic fitness, usually eliminating the exact population surplus, so that the original population size is restored. Selective removal can be either by truncation selection, probability selection, or partial truncation. To add biological realism, the user can specify a heritability of less than one, such that fitness variations caused by environmental noise will be added to the genetic fitness to establish the fitness phenotype, which is then the basis for selection. The individuals that survive selection will then be ready to repeat the cycle of mutation, reproduction, and selection.

During a single experiment, Mendel can routinely simulate hundreds of millions of newly arising mutations. Each mutation is tracked through all generations, until it is either lost or goes to fixation, or until the experiment is complete. Throughout the whole run Mendel is continuously monitoring, recording, and plotting the average number of mutations per individual, individual and average fitness, population size history, the fitness distributions of accumulating mutations, selection threshold histories, linkage block net fitness values, and mutant allele frequencies.

3. Forward-time population genetic numerical simulations

There are numerous forward-time simulation tools currently in use within the field of population genetics. Detailed reviews on the subject are available elsewhere (e.g., see Carvajal-Rodgríguez, 2008; Kim & Wiehe, 2008; Liu et al., 2008; Carvajal-Rodríguez, 2010). It is useful to provide a general overview of these programs to properly appreciate the types of problems that can be addressed with such simulations. Every forward-time simulation is designed with a particular application in mind, and each is best suited to study a certain class of scenarios.

3.1 FPG

The FPG (forward population genetic) simulation is the most similar to Mendel in concept (Hey, 2009). The user is able to define a mutation rate per generation for deleterious, neutral, and beneficial mutations, a fitness model (i.e., whether mutations combine additively, multiplicatively, or epistatically), a population size (i.e., number of genomes), and various other parameters. It is possible to track average fitness over time and perform analyses for linkage disequilibrium, fitness, and heterozygosity at the conclusion of an experiment. However, FPG is not readily accessible to most biologists. Running the program requires the user to understand and construct a string of input values at the command line level. Some of these values are not intuitive, e.g., a populational selection coefficient. FPG is also limited in terms of genome and population sizes. Its distributed version allows only 1000 sequences, and each sequence is restricted to 32 polymorphic sites, limiting the total number of effective mutations to 32000. This may be sufficient to model some long-term dynamics of populations with very small genomes, but it is generally inadequate for eukaryotic organisms. Finally, when large numbers of mutations occur, FPG appears to ignore fixed mutations after the fitness exceeds what can be stored as a floating point. Thus this program appears to ignore fixed mutations and their fitness effects to save computational resources, sometimes leading to counterintuitive output. Because of these considerations, FPG may work well for simple illustrative case studies but simply cannot handle the population sizes and number of mutations necessary to realistically address most biological scenarios. Perhaps its greatest limitation is that it models all mutations within a class (e.g., deleterious) as having identical fitness effects.

3.2 SimuPOP

SimuPOP is another forward-time simulation well-suited for tackling problems that involve a small number of functional loci. This program is especially helpful when studying the evolutionary dynamics of disease predisposing alleles. SimuPOP also allows the user to define auxiliary information for individual organisms. This information can be used to group organisms into virtual subpopulations, potentiating assortative mating based on characteristics such as genotype, sex, or age. Though flexible, simuPOP is challenging to use. Perhaps one of its largest drawbacks is that the user must write a Python macro to run an experiment. This can be an arduous task for even modestly complex evolutionary scenarios, as it requires a deep understanding of simuPOP and how to utilize its various components.

3.3 FREGENE

FREGENE is most innovative not so much for its novel implementation and flexibility, but rather for its use of a rescaling technique to make large problems less computationally intensive. Specifically, both population size (N) and number of generations are decreased by a factor of $\lambda > 1$, while all rate parameters (e.g., mutation, recombination, and migration rates) are increased by the same factor. This can be relaxed at the end of an experiment, such that (for example) the population size expands linearly from N/λ to N. Though this is clearly more computationally expedient than modeling full populations for full lengths of time, it is not ideal. For example, many processes depend on the absolute (not scaled) parameters, such as the fixation probability of beneficial mutations (Kim & Wiehe, 2008). Moreover, more advanced simulation software can usually handle the true population sizes and rates of interest, so there is often no need for such rescaling. FREGENE also implements an uncommon distribution of mutational fitness effects, drawing selection coefficients from two normal distributions (one each for deleterious and beneficial mutations) with user-specified means and variances. This is also sub-optimal, as it has long been agreed that the distribution of mutational fitness effects is approximately exponential, such that the majority of effective mutations are relatively low-impact (Eyre-Walker & Keightley, 2007).

3.4 Forwsim

Forwsim is another tool that implements a novel technique to save computational resources. To do this, the user can ask the simulation to look k generations ahead in order to determine which chromosomes will be passed to future generations. Once it is determined which chromosomes cannot contribute to future generations, those chromosomes are no longer simulated. Though there is a computational trade-off between looking k generations ahead and precluding the copying of unnecessary chromosomes, this process does serve to make many evolutionary scenarios more manageable. However, as previously stated, such techniques are often no longer necessary.

3.5 Avida

Finally, it is useful to contrast forward-time numerical simulations with digital life programs, especially the Avida simulation (Lenski et al., 2003; Ofria & Wilke, 2004), an elaboration of Tierra (Ray, 1991). There are important differences between the digital life approach and the numerical simulation approach described here. Forward-time numerical simulations attempt to simulate biological processes primarily by tracking numerical values (e.g., fitness) that change based on user-specified conditions. Using values measured in biological research (e.g., mutational fitness effects), the goal of numerical simulation is to accurately predict various populational dynamics under those conditions. A distribution of mutational fitness effects is specified, mutations are assigned certain locations on chromosomes, and their fitness effects simply increment or decrement an organism's fitness according to the selection model and gene interaction. Digital life, on the other hand, attempts to instantiate a model genome itself in the form of self-replicating computer code. Fitness then becomes an emergent value according to that program's behavior in the software environment. A full distribution of mutational fitness effects cannot be specified, only observed. In the case of Tierra, whatever changes allow the program to replicate faster in the simulated environment will be beneficial. Programs tend to shrink, allowing quicker self-replication, and parasitic behavior also emerges.

Avida builds on the concept of Tierra by introducing an external fitness function. In practice, this means that the Avida environment continually examines the population of digital organisms for certain computational operations. When these operations arise, the lucky organism can be rewarded with the ability to execute additional genomic instructions, allowing it to execute its code, and thus replicate, faster. The size of a reward is decided by the user, and experimental results depend critically on these values (Nelson & Sanford, 2011). It should be kept in mind that these operations are arbitrary, i.e., they only increase fitness because the programmer has imposed an arbitrary rule with fitness rewards. In other words, while genome shrinkage is a genuine way to increase replication speed, the fitness rewards based on certain computational operations can occur only because the programmer has altered the software environment to implement such a scheme.

Experiments with digital life systems are usually conducted with the goal of shedding light on general principles that are relevant to all self-replicating systems. However, though digital life research has produced a large number of publications in the biological literature, it appears to lack the ability to address the real issues in the genomics era. For example, genomes in Avida - only 50 to 100 monomers - are many orders of magnitude smaller than real biological genomes, and each Avida "mutation" which introduces a complete computational operation is assigned an unreasonably large fitness effect (i.e., 1.0 - 31.0; see Nelson & Sanford, 2011). Because mutations have an essential role in terms of introducing novel genetic variation, it is critical to simulate mutations realistically, and to examine realistically large genomes in which the fate of multiple low-impact mutations can be studied. The majority of fixations over the course of evolution do not involve highly beneficial mutations, but rather primarily involve nearly-neutral mutations (e.g., see Kimura, 1983; Hughes, 2008), so the biological relevance of digital life appears extremely limited.

It should now be clear that population genetics is more than an academic exercise. Many real-world problems that are informed by population genetics need resolution and demand biological models that honestly reflect nature. For example, there is very strong evidence that the human population is experiencing a marked decline in fitness due to the accumulation of very slightly deleterious mutations in both the mitochondrial and nuclear genomes (e.g., see Muller, 1950; Kondrashov, 1995; Loewe, 2006; Lynch, 2010). Thus there is a genuine need for serious and honest numerical simulations that can enable us to study these types of real-world problems. Specifically, it is imperative that we have the ability to model and calculate the net fitness effects of large numbers of low-impact mutations in large genomes.

Tool	Organisms & Populations	Mutation	Fitness & Selection
Avida (C++) Lenski et al., 2003; Ofria & Wilke, 2004; Nelson & Sanford, 2011	Organisms (typically asexual and haploid) contain genomes comprised of machine code instructions, as well as stacks and registers for storing and manipulating numbers. Populations exist on a two dimensional grid.	Mutations randomly substitute, insert, or delete one of 26 machine code instructions in the genome. The user specifies the various mutation rates.	Organisms replace each other when they produce a daughter cell. Speed of replication determines fitness, and this can be increased by either genome shrinkage or rewards for computational tasks.
Forwsim (C++) Padhukasahasram et al., 2008	Diploid organisms contain chromosome arrays that store the locations of mutations. The user specifies a probability of selfing. Populations of constant size reproduce with non-overlapping generations.	Mutations occur at a Poisson-distributed rate and insert new integers into chromosome arrays, which may undergo recombination. The number of sites is finite, but mutations occur only at non-polymorphic sites. Locations which are no longer polymorphic are removed.	If using natural selection, the evolution of selected and neutral sites is carried out separately, with selected sites considered first. The program excels at simulating genetic drift in a standard Wright-Fisher process.
FPG (C) Hey, 2009	Diploid organisms contain a user-defined number of chromosomes with a user-specified number of segments. Each segment can hold 32 mutations. It is possible to specify subpopulations. Populations of constant size reproduce with non-overlapping generations.	The user specifies one mutational fitness effect; deleterious and beneficial mutations have equal but opposite effects. Dominance and epistasis are user-specified. No segregating site in the population can receive another mutation. A maximum of 32,000 mutations can be tracked.	The user specifies a fitness model (additive, multiplicative, or epistatic). If fitness falls below a certain point, fixed mutations are ignored thereafter.

Tool	Organisms & Populations	Mutation	Fitness & Selection
FREGENE (C++) Hoggart et al., 2007; Chadeau-Hyam et al., 2008	Sexual diploid organisms (specified selfing probability). Genomes are single linear sequences represented as lists of sites at which a minor allele is present. Genomes recombine. Allows subpopulations. Populations of constant size reproduce with non-overlapping generations.	Deleterious and beneficial mutational fitness effects are modeled as two user-specified normal distributions. Two allele, finite sites model. Dominance, heritability, and recombination are also user-specified. Mutations occur independently at a constant rate. After a derived allele reaches fixation, it no longer affects fitness.	The user defines loci to be under selection, and can restrict such selection to subpopulations or time periods. Individual fitness is equal to unity plus the sum of contributions of selected sites.
Mendel's Accountant (Fortran 90) Sanford et al., 2007	Organisms (typically sexual diploid; selfing is user-specified) contain a user-defined number of chromosomes with a user-specified number of linkage blocks. Allows subpopulations. Populations of constant size reproduce with non-overlapping generations.	Mutations occur at a Poisson-distributed rate with Weibull-distributed fitness effects. Proportions of deleterious and beneficial mutations are user-specified. Allows heritability, dominance, and recombination. Infinite sites, infinite allele model, though back mutations may be specified.	The user selects a fitness model (additive, multiplicative, or epistatic). The user also sets the reproduction rate, with a higher reproduction rate allowing more intense selection (population size must be maintained). All loci may incur mutations affecting fitness.
SimuPOP (Python)	User defines ploidy, number of chromosomes, and loci under selection. The user chooses a mating scheme (including random mating and selfing). Allows subpopulations. Individual information can be specified, e.g., age, allowing non-random mating.	User-defined loci are used to store mutations, represented in a genome by sequential non-negative numbers. Implements a finite sites k-allele model, but allows other models to be specified.	The user specifies a fitness model (multiplicative, additive, or hetergenous). Fitness is assigned to individuals before mating, and parents to reproduce are chosen with probabilities proportional to their fitness.

Table 1. Comparison of several available population genetic simulations.

Readers are encouraged to examine these and other programs to determine which is best suited for particular applications (Carvajal-Rodgríguez, 2008; Kim & Wiehe, 2008; Liu et al., 2008; Carvajal-Rodríguez, 2010). Among these forward-time simulations, Mendel appears to be unique in that it is the first comprehensive (and hence most biologically realistic) population genetics numerical simulator. Mendel can simultaneously consider nearly all of the major factors that are recognized to be operational in a real population, and yields a multi-dimensional view of how populations really change. Moreover, the user has an intuitive and user-friendly interface, such that the user need only specify desired values for all available parameters. Mendel was designed and implemented in Fortran 90 to optimize use of computer resources, which allows the user to use an ordinary laptop computer to track many millions of mutations - orders of magnitude more than would be possible with any other application currently available. Very significantly, Mendel for the first time gives us the ability to model the net fitness effects of large numbers of low-impact mutations in large genomes.

Although Mendel is undergoing continuous enhancement, it has already demonstrated its ability to address a wide range of biological questions. Mendel is open-source code, and researchers are welcome to use it as a spring-board for further improvement. Mendel would seem to provide the most logical platform for building even more advanced simulators, which may eventually enable us to test essentially any biological scenario.

4. Applications

We briefly summarize below some basic findings already observed in various comprehensive numerical simulation applications. Some of these findings were exactly as would have been expected, while other findings seemed very surprising (although, upon reflection, they are clearly logical and correct).

4.1 Deleterious mutation accumulation

Mendel keeps a tally of how many deleterious mutations have accumulated in each individual. Mendel very consistently shows us that the mean deleterious mutation count per individual increases at an approximately constant rate over time (Sanford et al., 2007b; Gibson et al., 2012). This appears to be a very fundamental phenomenon (Figure 1). In fact, we can only simulate a substantially non-linear accumulation of deleterious mutation count per individual by using highly artificial parameters (Figure 2; see Brewer et al., 2012). Specifically, to cause mutation count per individual to plateau requires all deleterious mutations to have approximately equal affects on fitness, full or partial truncation selection, and sexual recombination. This combination of conditions is highly improbable under most natural circumstances. For example, organisms with very small genomes such as viruses should have a relatively narrow range of mutational fitness effects, but such organisms generally lack any type of regular sexual recombination. The general problem of ever-increasing genetic load within natural populations represents a widely recognized evolutionary paradox (Kondrashov, 1995; Crow, 1997; Sanford et al., 2007b; Gibson et al., 2012) and requires more research. Biologically realistic numerical simulations are the only practical means to further elucidate this problem, because the problem involves high numbers of very low-impact mutations, biological noise, and selection interference.

4.2 Beneficial mutation accumulation

Mendel also keeps a tally of how many beneficial mutations have accumulated in each individual. Like deleterious mutations, the number of beneficial mutations per individual tends to increase at a relatively constant rate, except for a very small class of beneficial mutations that have relatively large effects on fitness. Above a certain fitness effect, beneficial mutations are strongly amplified, leading to a period of accelerated mutation accumulation for that set of mutations and any mutations linked to them. The rapid amplification of high-impact beneficial mutations is as would be as expected, but it is striking to see that the large majority of beneficial mutations are too subtle to respond to

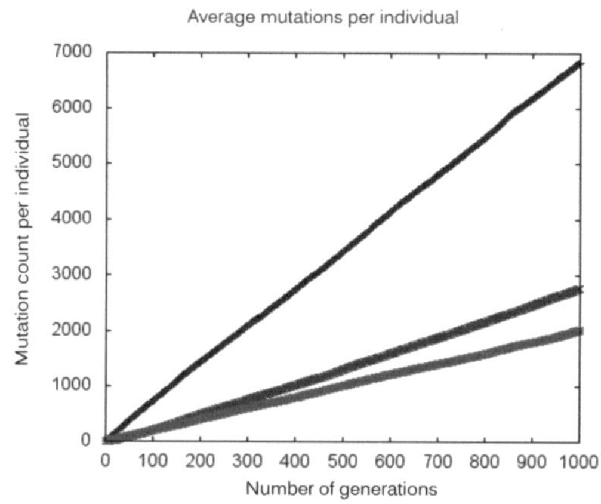

Fig. 1. Mutation accumulation in Mendel. Comprehensive numerical simulation reveals that mutation accumulation over time is largely linear. Mean mutation count per individual was tracked during the course of a Mendel experiment using default settings, except that selection efficiency was optimized (fitness heritability = 1, truncation selection). Input mutations were 10% beneficial, 20% neutral, and 70% deleterious. In this experiment, mean fitness increased by 210%. As can be seen, all three classes of mutation accumulated essentially linearly, but differed relative to their rate of accumulation (slope). Neutral mutations accumulated as expected, just as if there were no selection (bottom line). The deleterious mutations accumulated slightly slower than would be expected if there were no selection (upper line). The beneficial mutations accumulated almost 3 times faster than would be expected if there were no selection (middle line).

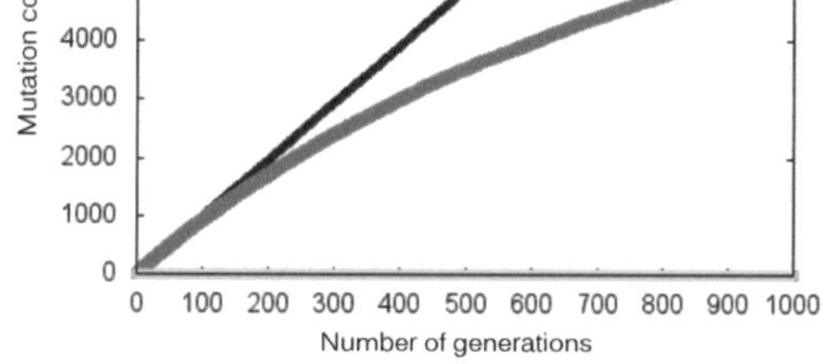

Fig. 2. The effects of uniform fitness effects on deleterious mutation accumulation. Only highly unrealistic conditions cause deleterious mutation accumulation to significantly diverge from linearity (such that deleterious mutation count per individual begins to plateau). The straight line reflects an experiment employing the basic Mendel default settings but with all mutations being deleterious (a broad distribution of mutation fitness effects, fitness heritability = 0.2, probability selection). The curved line reflects the same run but where all mutations had an equal fitness effect (-.0001) and truncation selection was employed.

selection (Sanford et al., 2012). Except for those few high-impact beneficial mutations which are strongly amplified, the ratio of beneficial versus deleterious mutations does not change dramatically in response to selection (see Figures 1 and 3). Since it is well known that deleterious mutations arise much more frequently than do beneficial mutations, this means that many more functional nucleotide sites are being disrupted than are being established, even with intense selection. This suggests there should be a strong natural tendency toward net loss of genetic information over time, even while a limited number of beneficial mutations are being strongly amplified. This represents a second major evolutionary paradox that demands serious attention by researchers. Again, it seems clear that this problem can best be understood by further numerical simulation experiments.

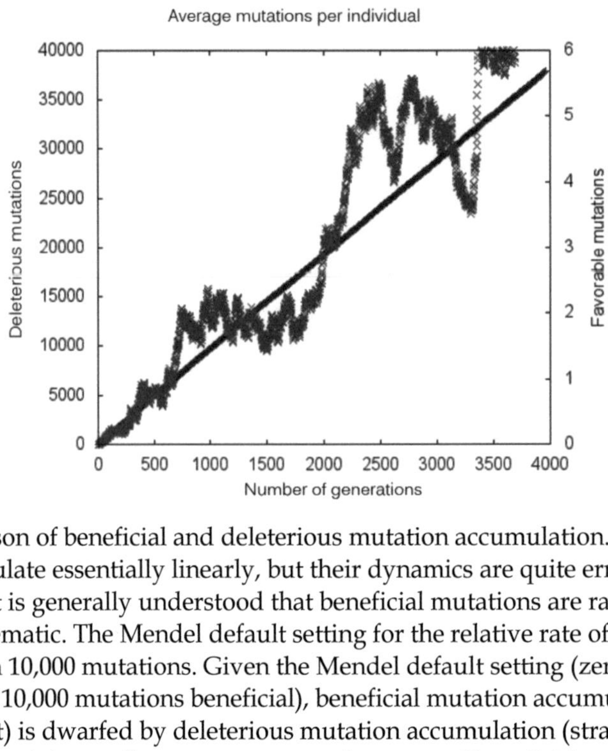

Fig. 3. A comparison of beneficial and deleterious mutation accumulation. Beneficial mutations accumulate essentially linearly, but their dynamics are quite erratic due to their rare occurrence. It is generally understood that beneficial mutations are rare, which makes their study problematic. The Mendel default setting for the relative rate of beneficial mutation is one in 10,000 mutations. Given the Mendel default setting (zero neutral mutations, one in 10,000 mutations beneficial), beneficial mutation accumulation (jagged line, scale on right) is dwarfed by deleterious mutation accumulation (straight line, scale on left). For this reason it is usually necessary to employ rates of beneficial mutation which are exaggerated by several orders of magnitude in order to study the behavior of this class of mutation in detail.

4.3 Change in mean fitness over time

Mendel continuously computes the mean fitness of the population based upon the mutation content of each individual. Mendel reveals that populations tend to decline in fitness (due to the continuous accumulation of deleterious mutations), except when there is a sufficiently high rate of beneficial mutations with sufficiently high fitness effects (Figure 4). There is a critical point where beneficial mutations are both frequent enough and have a strong enough fitness impact to allow stabilization of population fitness. Above this critical point, mean fitness can then increase very rapidly. This raises a variety of interesting research problems. For example, what conditions are required to reach this critical point needed for fitness stabilization? It appears that when mean fitness is increasing due to just a few high-impact mutations at a few chromosomal locations, a much larger number of functional nucleotides are being disrupted due to relatively low-impact deleterious mutations. The latter are genetically linked to the former in the vast majority of cases. Does this mean that the functional genome size is continuously shrinking? How might we simulate selection for traits which require many beneficial mutations, but none of which are beneficial or selectable apart from the others? How might the multitude of functional, but low-impact, nucleotides in a genome arise? All these questions can best be addressed using comprehensive numerical simulation.

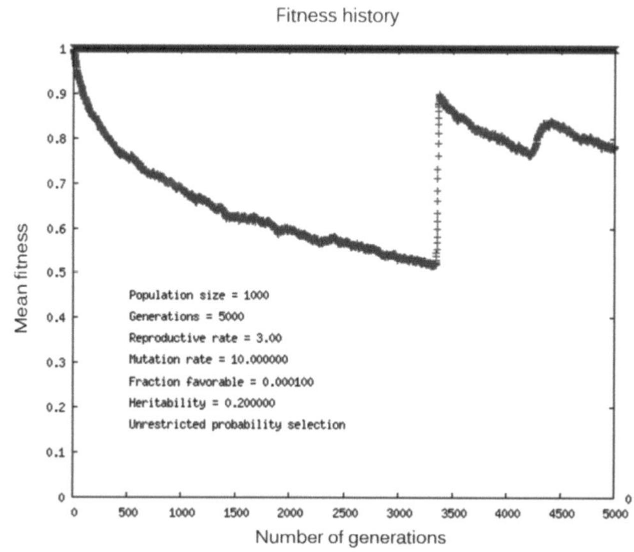

Fig. 4. Fitness trajectory and high-impact beneficial mutations. Change in a population's mean fitness is determined by the net effect of a large number of low-impact deleterious mutations and a small number of relatively high-impact beneficial mutations. In this experiment Mendel's default settings were used (beneficial mutation rate = 0.0001), except that beneficial fitness effects were allowed to range up to 1.0 (one such mutation would double fitness). In 5000 generations the mean deleterious mutation count per individual was 47,648, while the mean beneficial mutation count per individual was 9.8. As can be seen, just two high-impact beneficial mutations largely compensated for over 40,000 deleterious mutations.

4.4 Selection threshold

Mendel's Accountant enables the empirical determination of the "selection threshold" of a given population, which is quantified using a newly proposed statistic, ST. The selection threshold concept is key to understanding the big picture regarding the actual capabilities and limitations of natural selection within a given population. A population's selection threshold is an emergent property of a population and its exact circumstances. It is the consequence of the net effect of all those variables that enhance or interfere with selection efficacy. One of the primary variables that limits selection efficacy is the phenomenon of selection interference, wherein selection for one mutation interferes with selection for other mutations. This phenomenon has been recognized for a long time, but has until now eluded quantification.

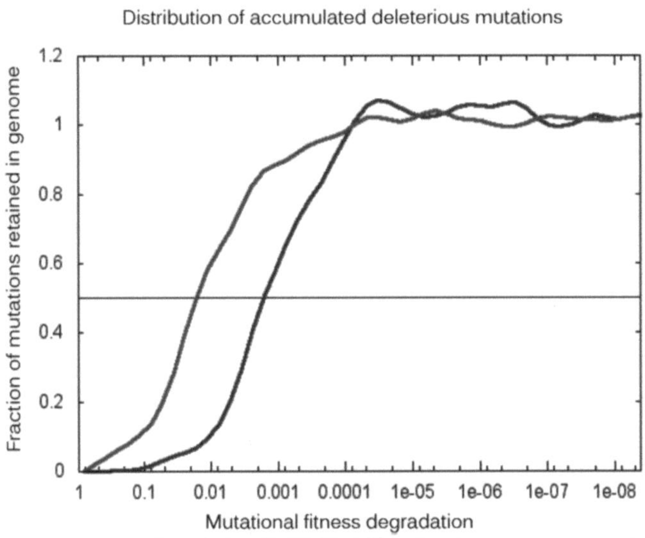

Fig. 5. The effects of fitness effect on mutation accumulation. Selection breaks down for most low-impact deleterious mutations. In this Mendel experiment, 80% of all mutations were made recessive (with 5% expression in the heterozygotic state) and 20% were made dominant (95% expression in the heterozygotic state). The rate of deleterious mutation accumulation (y axis) ranged from zero (no accumulation) to one (accumulation as if no selection). Mutational fitness effect is shown on the x-axis (log scale). As can be seen, deleterious mutations with very high impacts are selectively eliminated very effectively, but mutations with very low impacts are not affected by selection at all. The selection threshold (where the accumulation curve intersects 0.5, shown with a straight line) is where mutations are accumulating at half the rate they would in the absence of selection. In this experiment, the selection threshold is about one order of magnitude higher (curve to left) for recessive than for dominant mutations (curve to right). A similar selection threshold can be plotted for beneficial mutations.

The selection threshold value for deleterious mutations (ST_d) is defined as the mutational fitness effect at which mutations accumulate at exactly half the rate as would occur if there were no selection (Figure 5). By parity of reasoning, the selection threshold value for beneficial mutations (ST_b) is defined as the mutational fitness effect at which mutations accumulate at twice the rate as would occur if there were no selection (not shown). Mendel continuously monitors these selection threshold values during an experiment. We observe that the selection threshold is initially very high in all experiments, but drops dramatically in the first several hundred generations, and eventually approaches a (minimum) equilibrium value. The amount of time required to reach this "selection equilibrium" is strongly affected by population size, with large populations requiring deep time to reach their full selection potential (minimal selection threshold).

Selection threshold values are, to our knowledge, the only available diagnostic of how effectively selection can operate under a specific set of circumstances, in terms of eliminating bad mutations and amplifying good mutations. It is worth noting that Kimura's (1983) well-known inequality, $|s| \leq 1/(2N_e)$, is an attempt to estimate the selection threshold based upon the random noise inherent in finite population sizes alone. However, many other parameters affect the efficacy of selection, including the mutation rate, the distribution of mutational fitness effects, environmental noise, mode of selection, and others. The final outcome of an experiment largely hinges on the emergent selection threshold values. This statistic is the best means to bring together all the "pieces of the population puzzle," enabling researchers to gauge the long-term genetic health of a population. A low threshold value should reflect a healthy population, allowing selection to "see" more low-impact mutations, while a high threshold value will reflect a population that is at risk of on-going genetic deterioration due to "selection breakdown" for most (low-impact) nuceotide positions in the genome.

4.5 Net effect of linkage blocks

We know that chromosomes do not recombine uniformly, but have recombinational hotspots, which sub-divide each chromosome into numerous "linkage blocks". There is little recombination within a linkage block, so mutations that arise within the same linkage block will tend to be transmitted linked together indefinitely, from generation to generation. Mendel models this in a biologically realistic way, so that the effects of the linked mutations can be studied. This opens the way to study the phenomenon of "Muller's Ratchet" as it applies to individual linkage blocks. Mendel also allows the examination of the relative abundance of linkage blocks which have a net fitness gain versus a net fitness loss (Figure 6).

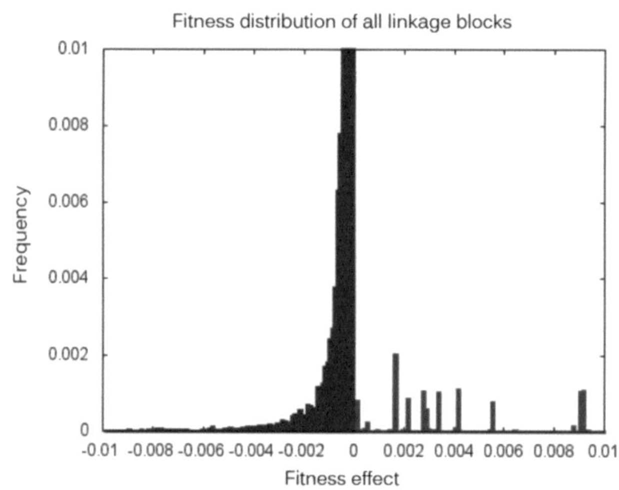

Fig. 6. The net fitness effects of linkage blocks reflect the distribution of accumulating mutations. This Mendel experiment employed the default parameters, except 20% of mutations were neutral, 1% were beneficial, and the maximal beneficial fitness effect was .01. Fitness was nearly stable and rising gradually. Linkage blocks with a net deleterious fitness effect are shown left of center, while linkage blocks with a net beneficial effect are shown right of center. As can be seen, almost all linkage blocks had a net effect which was modestly deleterious. Only 1.7% of all linkage blocks had a net beneficial effect, but that net beneficial effect was usually substantial.

4.6 Population bottlenecks

In nature, populations routinely go through bottlenecks in population size. It has been proposed that this might be biologically useful in terms of genetically homogenizing a population. It has even been proposed that regular downward fluctuations in population size might help "pump out" or purge a population's deleterious mutations. We have used Mendel to study episodes of population size contraction in mature populations, and we have observed that any episode that even marginally reduces total genetic variation simultaneously causes irreversible genetic damage. This is seen as a substantial fitness decline that does not fully recover when population size returns to normal, and which corresponds to an increased rate of fixation of deleterious mutations and an elevated deleterious selection threshold (Figure 7). It appears that it is very problematic to achieve homogenization of a mature out-crossing population by bottlenecking without risking population extinction. We have also used Mendel to examine cyclic bottlenecking. We observe that this does not "pump out" deleterious mutations, but rather "pumps in" such mutations due to elevated selection thresholds during each population contraction and a correspondingly higher rate of fixation of deleterious alleles.

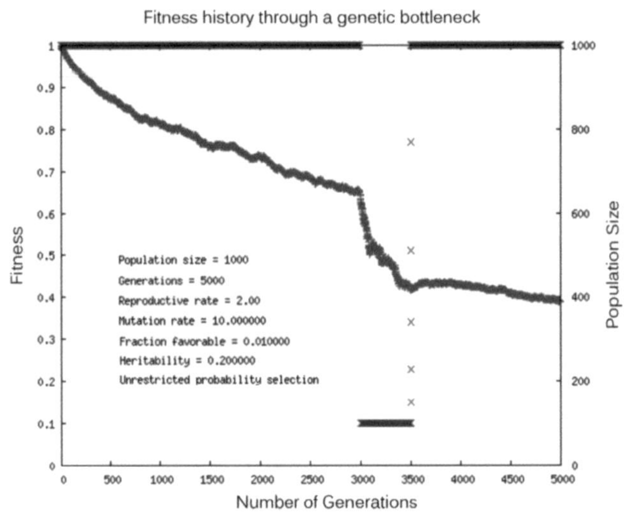

Fig. 7. The effects of population bottlenecks on average fitness. Population bottlenecks sufficient to have any noticeable impact cause irreversible genetic damage in out-crossing species. In this Mendel experiment, 1% of all mutations were beneficial, with the maximal beneficial fitness effect being .01. Eighty percent of mutations were recessive. After 3000 generations, population size was reduced from 1000 to 100 for 500 generations, after which population size was allowed to expand, restoring the population size (top line) to 1000 (scale on right). As can be seen, during the bottleneck fitness declined roughly 30% and failed to recover substantially when population size was restored.

4.7 Allele frequencies

Mendel tracks allele frequencies. This allows the study of the rate of polymorphism (alleles with a frequency of more than 1%), and the rate of fixation (alleles with frequencies over

99%). As expected, Mendel shows that the vast majority of new alleles are lost by drift while they are still very rare. We see that the maximal number of polymorphic alleles is primarily limited by population size and population sub-structure (i.e., sub-populations that seldom inter-mate). Likewise, rate of fixation is profoundly affected by population size and population sub-structure. The rate of fixation is extremely slow except for relatively high-impact beneficial mutations, which can fix quite rapidly - in just hundreds of generations. Surprisingly, we routinely see that under the most biologically realistic conditions, many more deleterious mutations go to fixation than do beneficial mutations (because they arise at a much higher rate; Figure 8). Much more work remains to be done to better understand the determinants of polymorphism frequencies and rates of fixation.

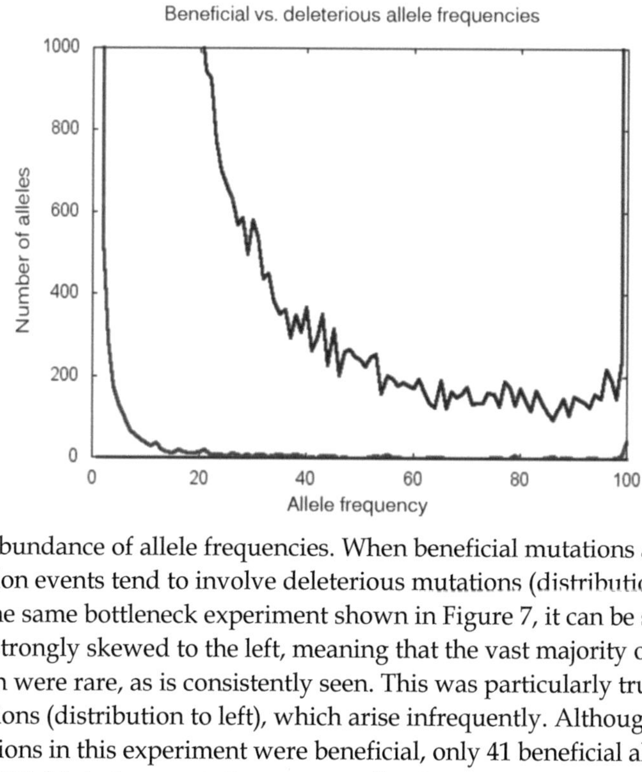

Fig. 8. Relative abundance of allele frequencies. When beneficial mutations are rare, the vast majority of fixation events tend to involve deleterious mutations (distribution to right). Drawing from the same bottleneck experiment shown in Figure 7, it can be seen that allele frequencies are strongly skewed to the left, meaning that the vast majority of alleles present in the population were rare, as is consistently seen. This was particularly true in the case of beneficial mutations (distribution to left), which arise infrequently. Although a generous 1% of all new mutations in this experiment were beneficial, only 41 beneficial alleles went to fixation, while 9327 deleterious mutations went to fixation.

4.8 Sexual reproduction

Much has been said about the biological importance of sexual recombination. This can most clearly be seen by using numerical simulation to contrast deleterious mutation accumulation in a normal sexual popuation and an identical population that reproduces asexually (Figure 9). The difference is very dramatic; the asexual population undergoes genetic degeneration very rapidly and the decline in fitness is distictly linear, while in the sexual population, the fitness decline is modest and approximates exponential decay. These findings confirm expectation, because it has long been known that the absence of recombination in asexual genomes causes a gravely deterministic decay in fitness known as Muller's ratchet (e.g., see Loewe, 2006).

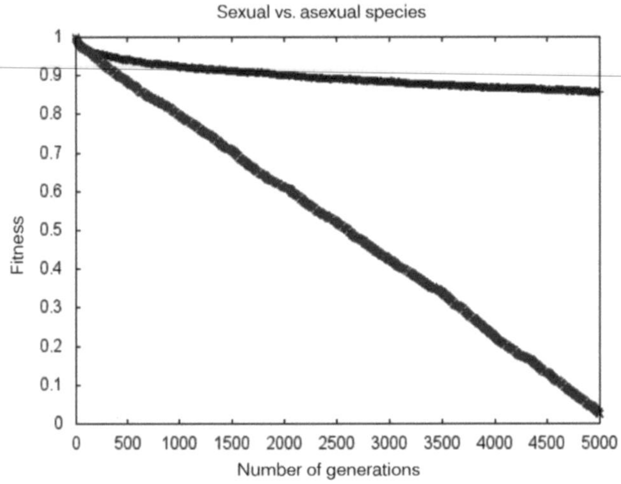

Fig. 9. The effects of sexual reproduction on fitness decline. Asexual populations are subject to disastrous fitness decline due to Muller's Ratchet. A Mendel experiment with default settings (except truncation selection was employed) was compared to the same run where reproduction was clonal, i.e., without sexual recombination. The upper line represents the first run using the default settings, resulting in a relatively modest level of fitness decline. The lower line represents the second run where sexual recombination was turned off, resulting in a rapid and very linear decline in fitness, causing extinction in just over 5000 generations.

4.9 Future developments

In addition to the features and applications described above, other Mendel features recently developed or still under development include simulation of: a) synergistic epistasis; b) group selection; c) selection for altruistic traits; and d) analysis of specific sets of mutations that any user may upload into a population prior to simulation. Mendel is being modified to be compatible with most computer environments. Hopefully many researchers will use this program as a platform to develop far superior numerical simulations.

5. Conclusion

It is clear that there is great utility in comprehenisve numerical simulations, becaue they alone allow us to examine – simultaneously – the many elements of a given population's dynamics. Not only does this mean we can finally get an integrated "big picture" view of how a population changes, but we can use the same program to examine the same population in great detail from many specific vantage points. In light of the examples summarized above, it is clear there are numerous research problems which cannot be adequately addressed without comprehensive numerical simulation tools.

6. Acknowledgments

This work was supported in part by the FMS Foundation and by Rainbow Technololgies, Inc.

7. References

Brewer, W.; Baumgardner, J. & Sanford, J. (2012). Using Numerical Simulation to Test the "Mutation-Count" Hypothesis, In: *Biological Information – New Perspectives* (in press).

Carvajal-Rodríguez, A. (2008). Simulation of Genomes: A Review. *Current Genomics*, Vol. 9, (May 2008), pp. 155-159.

Carvajal-Rodríguez, A. (2010). Simulation of Genes and Genomes Forward in Time. *Current Genomics*, Vol. 11, (March 2010), pp. 58-61.

Chadeau-Hyam, M.; Hoggart, C.J.; O'Reilly, P.F.; Whittaker, J.C.; De Iorio, M. & Balding, D.J. (2008). Fregene: Simulation of Realistic Sequence-Level Data in Populations and Ascertained Samples. *BMC Bioinformatics*, Vol. 9, (September 2008), p. 364.

Crow, J.F. (1997). The High Spontanoues Mutation Rate: Is it Health Risk? *Proceedings of the National Academy of Sciences USA*, Vol. 94, (August 1997), pp. 8380-8386.

Eyre-Walker, A. & Keightley, P.D. (2007). The Distribution of Fitness Effects of New Mutations. *Nature Reviews Genetics*, Vol. 8, (August 2007), pp. 610-618.

Gibson, P.; Baumgardner, J.; Brewer, W. & Sanford, J. (2012). Can Biological Information Be Sustained By Purifying Natural Selection? In: *Biological Information – New Perspectives* (in press).

Hey, J. (2009). FPG - A Computer Program For Forward Population Genetic Simulation, 20.07.2011, Available from http://lifesci.rutgers.edu/~heylab/ProgramsandData/Programs/FPG/FPG_Documentation.htm

Hoggart, C.J.; Chadeau-Hyam, M.; Clark T.G.; Lampariello, R.; Whittaker, J.C.; De Iorio, M. & Blading, D.J. (2007). Sequence-Level Population Simulations Over Large Genomic Regions. *Genetics*, Vol. 177, (November 2007), pp. 1725-1731.

Hughes, A.L. (2008). Near Neutrality: Leading Edge of the Neutral Theory of Molecular Evolution. *Annals of the New York Academy of Sciences*, Vol. 1133, (2008), pp. 162-179.

Kim, Y. & Wiehe, T. (2009). Simulation of DNA Sequence Evolution Under Models of Recent Directional Selection. *Briefings in Bioinformatics*, Vol. 10, (January 2009), pp. 84-96.

Kimura, M. (1983). *The Neutral Theory of Molecular Evolution*, Cambridge University Press, ISBN 0-521-31793-2, Cambridge.

Kondrashov, A.S. (1995). Contamination of the Genome by Very Slightly Deleterious Mutations: Why Have We Not Died 100 Times Over? *Journal of Theoretical Biology*, Vol. 175, (August 1995), pp. 583-594.

Lenski, R.E.; Ofria, C.; Pennock, R.T. & Adami, C. (2003). The Evolutionary Origin of Complex Features. *Nature*, Vol. 423, (May 2003), pp. 139-144.

Li, H. & Durbin, R. (2011). Inference of Human Population History From Individual Whole-Genome Sequences. *Nature*, Vol. 475, (July 2011), pp. 493-496.

Liu, Y.; Athanasiadis, G. & Weale, M.E. (2008). A Survey of Genetic Simulation Software For Populations and Epidemiological Studies. *Human Genomics*, Vol. 3, (September 2008), pp. 79-86.

Loewe, L. (2002). Evolution@home: Global Computing Quantifies Evolution Due To Muller's Ratchet. *BMC Bioinformatics*, Vol. 6, Suppl. 3, (September 2005), p. P18.

Loewe, L. (2006). Quantifying the Genomic Decay Paradox Due To Muller's Ratchet in Human Mitochondrial DNA. *Genetical Research*, Vol. 87, (April 2006), pp. 133-159.

Lynch, M. (2010). Rate, Molecular Spectrum, and Consequences of Human Mutation. *Proceedings of the National Academy of Sciences USA*, Vol. 107, No. 3, pp. 961-968.

Muller, H.J. (1950). Our Load of Mutations. *American Journal of Human Genetics*, Vol. 2, (1950), pp. 111-176.

Nelson, C.W. & Sanford, J.C. (2011). The Effects of Low-Impact Mutations in Digital Organisms. *Theoretical Biology and Medical Modelling*, Vol. 8, (April 2011), p. 9.

Ofria, C. & Wilke, C.O. (2004). Avida: A Software Platform for Research in Computational Evolutionary Biology. *Artificial Life*, Vol. 10, No. 2, (2004), pp. 191-229.

Padhukasahasram, B.; Marjoram, P.; Wall, J.D.; Bustamante, C.D. & Nordborg, M. (2008). Exploring Population Genetic Models With Recombination Using Efficient Forward-Time Simulations. *Genetics*, Vol. 178, (April 2008), pp. 2417-2427.

Peng, B. & Amos, C.I. (2008). Forward-Time Simulations of Nonrandom Mating Populations Using simuPOP. *Bioinformatics*, Vol. 24, (June 2008), pp. 1408-1409.

Peng, B. & Amos, C.I. (2010). Forward-Time Simulations of Realistic Samples For Genome-Wide Association Studies. *BMC Bioinformatics*, Vol. 11, (September 2010), p. 442.

Peng, B. & Kimmel, M. (2005). simuPOP: A Forward-Time Population Genetics Simulation Environment. *Bioinformatics*, Vol. 21, (September 2005), pp. 3686-3687.

Peng, B. & Liu, X. (2010). Simuating Sequences of the Human Genome with Rare Variants. *Human Heredity*, Vol. 70, (January 2010), pp. 287-291.

Ray, T.S. (1991). An Approach to the Synthesis of Life, In: *Artificial Life II, SFI Studies in the Sciences of Complexity, Vol. X: 1991*, Langton, C.G.; Taylor, C.; Farmer, J.D. & Rasmussen, S., (Eds.), pp. 371-408, Addison-Wesley, Redwood City, CA.

Sanford, J.; Baumgardner, J.; Brewer, W.; Gibson, P. & ReMine, W. (2007a). Mendel's Accountant: A Biologically Realistic Forward-Time Population Genetics Program. *Scalable Computing: Practice and Experience*, Vol. 8, No. 2, (2007), pp. 147-165.

Sanford, J.; Baumgardner, J.; Gibson, P.; Brewer, W. & ReMine, W. (2007b). Using Computer Simulation to Understand Mutation Accumulation Dynamics and Genetic Load, In: *7th International Conference on Computational Science, Proceedings, Part II, LCNS 4488: 2007*, Shi, Y.; van Albada, G.D.; Dongarra, J. & Sloot, P.M.A., (Eds.), pp. 386-392, Springer-Verlag, Beijing, China.

Sanford, J.; Baumgardner, J. & Brewer, W. (2012). Selection Threshold Severely Constrains Capture of Beneficial Mutations, In: *Biological Information – New Perspectives* (in press).

Sauna, Z.E. & Kimchi-Sarfaty, C. (2011). Understanding the Contribution of Synonymous Mutations to Human Disease. *Nature Reviews Genetics*, Vol. 12, (October 2011), pp. 683-691.

Thorne, A.G. & Wolpoff, M.H. (1992). The Multiregional Evolution of Humans. *Scientific American*, Vol. 266, No. 4, (April 1992), pp. 76-83.

Wilson, A.C. & Cann, R.L. (1992). The Recent African Genesis of Humans. *Scientific American*, Vol. 266, No. 4, (April 1992), pp. 68-73.

8

Population Genetics in the Genomic Era

Shuhua Xu* and Wenfei Jin
Chinese Academy of Sciences Key Laboratory of Computational Biology,
Chinese Academy of Sciences and Max Planck Society (CAS-MPG)
Partner Institute for Computational Biology, Shanghai Institutes for Biological Sciences,
Chinese Academy of Sciences, Shanghai,
China

1. Introduction

Over the past decades, scientific research on population genetics has been facilitated greatly by advances in DNA genotyping and sequencing technologies, during which time it has transformed from a theory-driven field with little empirical data into a data-driven discipline with a deluge of data. The emergence of population genomics demarcated a transition from single-locus-based studies to genome-wide analyses of genetic variations, which benefits the identification of disease/trait associated genes and targets of natural selection. In particular, with the development of next-generation sequencing (NGS), a considerable number of individual genomes are becoming available. Nonetheless, the availability of genome-wide data not only is a big challenge for computational capability, which drives the statistics and methods to be more efficient, but also leads to some transitions on strategies and methodologies. For example, the traditional strategy for identifying targets of positive selection was based on candidate gene strategy that priori assumed a gene under selection and compared it with the null hypothesis. Genomic approaches, however, usually involve constructing an empirical distribution of a summary statistics across all loci, which quantifies a characteristic of the genetic variation, with the extreme tail of the distribution being defined as putative targets.

The analysis of genome-wide data has greatly improved our knowledge on mechanism of mutations and recombination, human origins and history, adaptation to local environment and variants underlying disease. However, some of these discoveries conflicted with the traditional views or models. For example, it is traditionally believed that beneficial mutation usually arises and increases in frequency to fixation, which was referred to as classic selective sweep model that almost all statistics detecting positive selection relied on, while recent genome-wide analysis showed that it was rarely the case in recent human evolution, which demands new models and statistics to depict and detect the signatures of positive selection. Meanwhile, great progress could be made by integrating these new discoveries to improve the mathematical models such as coalescent theory. In a nutshell, the advent of genomic data has influenced and will continue its influence on every corner of genetics, thus significantly accelerating the development of population genetics.

---

* Corresponding Author

Besides, genomic approach has also greatly facilitated the identification of diseases/traits associated genes. Genome-wide association studies (GWAS), genotyping millions of SNPs on thousands of individuals, has become a standard method in disease gene discovery in the past several years. However, the common variants identified by GWAS only account for a small fraction of the heritability thus fail to explain the majority of phenotypic variance in population. Therefore, as an alternative to the common disease common variants hypothesis (CDCV), several new hypotheses have been proposed.

In this chapter, we will focus only on those topics concerned with population genomics, i.e. methods, statistics and analysis based on high-density genome-wide data (either genotyping data or sequencing data), so the research category can be different from that of traditional population genetic studies relying on single locus or sparse loci.

2. Variation, recombination, haplotypes and inference of population parameters

2.1 Overview of genome-wide high-density data

Based on the current technologies and features, the genome-wide data can be roughly classified into genotyping data and sequencing data.

DNA Genotyping is the process of determining the status of DNA using biological assays and comparing it with known sequences. It is used either to track the alleles an individual inherited from his/her parents, or to reveal differentiations between individuals and populations. With most SNPs discovered in a small set of samples, the genotyping data have high proportion of SNPs with intermediate allele frequency. This ascertainment bias is likely to affect all statistics based on allele frequencies[1].

DNA Sequencing, on the other hand, includes several methods and technologies to determine the order of the nucleotides in DNA. The high demand for sequencing data has promoted the development of low-cost high-throughput sequencing technologies (also referred to as next-generation sequencing) that parallelize the sequencing process by producing thousands or millions of sequences at once[2]. These low-cost high-throughput technologies, including 454 Life Sciences (Roche) sequencing, Illumina Solexa sequencing, and Applied Biosystems SOLiD sequencing, will finally make the individual genomes affordable and accessible, initiating individual genomic era.

2.2 Genetic variations in human genome

Genetic variations refer to any genetic differences among individuals within one population or species, which provide the genetic basis of evolution. Since the nucleotide differentiation between individuals is estimated to be about 0.1%[3], meaning that there are about 3-million nucleotide differences between two unrelated individuals. The genetic variations in human genome can be classified into single nucleotide polymorphism (SNP), short insertion and deletion (indel), copy number variation (CNV), variable number tandem repeat (VNTR: including microsatellite and minisatellite), haplotype (including haplogroup), epigenetic and so on[4]. Among all these, SNP is a type of variation with one nucleotide differentiation in sequence, which is generally caused by single mutations, and it is estimated that there are about 30 million SNPs existing in human genomes, which makes them the most common genetic variations in human genomes.

There were various scientific endeavors for identifying the genetic variations after the completion of human genome project (HGP). For example, the International Haplotype Map Project (http://hapmap.ncbi.nlm.nih.gov) has provided the allele frequency of about 4 million SNPs in at least one population; the 1000 Genome Project is another international collaboration trying to provide the accurate haplotype information on all forms of human DNA polymorphism in multiple human populations, and the completion of its pilot phase has provided the location, allele frequency and local haplotype structure of ~15 million SNPs, 1 million indel and 20,000 structural variations, most of which being novel[5]. The sequencing data also showed that each individual cherished ~3 million variant SNPs, ~350,000 indel, 250-300 loss-of-function variants in annotated genes and 50-100 variants previously implicated in inherited disorders[5].

2.3 Linkage disequilibrium pattern and haplotype

In meiosis, one allele often transmits together with the alleles around it, which leads to association or correlation between loci close to each other, such phenomenon is called linkage disequilibrium (LD). The distribution of LD in human becomes a topic of great interest due to its fundamental role in gene mapping, recombination and human history[6]. Assuming two alleles A and B at two loci with frequencies π_A and π_B in the population, respectively, we expect the frequency of the AB haplotype to be $\pi_A\pi_B$ if the two loci are independent. If the frequency of AB haplotype in a population does not fit the following: $\pi_{AB} = \pi_A\pi_B$, the two loci are in LD. A wide variety of statistics have been proposed to measure LD, the simplest of which is $D = \pi_{AB}-\pi_A \pi_B$. Although D originates from the definition, its values are affected seriously by allele frequencies. Normalization of D is the most common way to address the dependence of D on marginal allele frequencies. Lewontin's D'[7, 8] , one of the normalized D, has the desirable property, and |D'| = 1 if there are only three gametic types or if two SNPs are in complete LD. Calculation of D' is:

$$D' = \begin{cases} \dfrac{D}{\min(\pi_A\pi_b, \pi_a\pi_B)} & D > 0 \\ \dfrac{D}{\min(\pi_A\pi_B, \pi_a\pi_b)} & D < 0 \end{cases}$$

where πa and πb are the allele frequencies of the alleles a and b, which are the counterpart of A and B in the same loci, respectively. The obvious drawback of D' is that its sampling properties are poorly understood when |D'| < 1. In addition, estimation of D' is strongly inflated in small samples, especially for rare variants. Currently, the most popular measure of LD between biallelic loci is r^2 (also referred to as Δ^2), whose values reflect the amount of information provided about each other:

$$r^2 = \frac{D^2}{\pi_A\pi_a\pi_B\pi_b}$$

In the case of $r^2 = 1$, which is known as perfect LD, it means the observation at one marker provides complete information about the other.

The completion of HapMap project has provided the fine-scale LD pattern of the human genome[9, 10]. First, it is found that LD varies remarkably on scales of 1-100kb, which are always discontinued and compose block-like structures. Second, haplotype diversity arises solely through mutation in the genome when recombine is absent. Thus SNPs arising on the same branch of the genealogy are in complete LD ($|D'| = 1$), while those happened on different branches have limited or no correlation. Third, although different populations have different haplotype frequencies, both common and rare haplotypes are usually shared among populations. Fourth, some SNPs located in recombination hotspots have very weak LD with neighboring SNPs, which is not well represented in tag SNPs. Finally, LD correlates with many genomic features such as recombination rate, mutation rate, G+C content, sequencing variation, repeat composition and chromosome length. A worldwide survey of haplotype and LD in the human genome showed that human history, to some extent, is reflected by the geographic distribution of haplotype, which looses diversity as distance increases from Africa[11].

2.4 Recombination in human population and its implication

By shaping the landscape of individual genomes per generation, recombination plays an important role in reproduction. However, it was not considered in the initial models of population genetics, which assumed that all loci are independent. In recent decades, LD pattern and haplotype pattern created by recombination have been realized harbored much information about recent population history, which has been extended to estimate population parameters and population history[12]. Despite the limited numbers of meioses in pedigree, the genetic map was reconstituted by counting crossover, which revealed the sex difference and recombination variation at megabase[13]. Sperm-typing studies on dozens of regions have demonstrated that most recombination events concentrated in very short regions of 1-2 kb, which are referred to as recombination hotspots with intensity from 4×10^{-4} cM to 0.14 cM[14].

Coalescent theory is a stochastic process that describes the distribution of underlying genealogic tree of individuals from idealized population[15]. When no recombination happened, the inheritance relationships of a group of samples can be represented by a genealogical tree, on which all samples are traced back to a single ancestral copy known as the most recent common ancestor (MRCA)[16], and differences of these samples on the tree are due to mutation events. However, recombination breaks up the chromosomes each generation and reduces LD, which increases haplotype diversity. Thus different regions on the genome may produce different trees due to recombination[17, 18]. If two loci are close to each other and recombination rarely occurred between them, the two trees are likely to be the same. However, as the genetic distance between the two loci increases, the correlation between the two trees decreases[17]. Therefore, a simple genealogic tree may not fully represent the ancestry of the sample of recombined chromosome. Instead, the complex graph[19], which includes a series of coalescence and recombination events, was proposed to represent the recombined chromosome, allowing us to recover the marginal genealogy at any given position[20]. The coalescent that integrated recombination was often referred to as the ancestral recombination graph (ARG)[18, 19], which benefits us a lot in understanding the effect of recombination. By considering where coalescent, recombination and mutation happened on the tree, we are able to infer the impact of recombination on patterns of genetic variation. On the other hand, if the procedure that generates the graph can be modeled, it is also possible for us to estimate the population parameters such as recombination rates[20].

2.5 Estimating recombination rates based on population genetic methods

On one hand, traditional pedigree studies generally do not provide fine-scale recombination rates due to the limited numbers of meioses in a few generations[13, 21]. On the other hand, sperm-typing analysis is extremely laborious and expensive despite its high-resolution[22]. Therefore, with the availability of a deluge of SNP data, statistical inferences of recombination rates using population genetic methods become the major strategy to obtain the landscape of fine-scale recombination. The simplest and most direct way to identify the historical recombination events is to analyze the closest pair-wise SNPs, which, however, does not model the recombination process and recombination graph. For examples, we assume two bi-allelic loci with ancestral and derived allele A/B and a/b, respectively, and all potential haplotypes constituted by the two loci are AB, Ab, aB, ab. For infinite sites mutation model, recombination must have occurred in history when all of these haplotypes were found[20]. Performing four-gamete test (FGT) on all pairs of loci in a region can identify the intervals at which recombination occurred. Assuming all recombination originated from the same recombination event, R_m conservatively estimated the minimum number of recombination that had occurred in history[20], which would underestimate the real recombination events[23].

To overcome the shortcoming of counting recombination events directly, it is necessary to model the underlying recombination process. The coalescent that integrated recombination was often referred to as the ancestral recombination graph (ARG)[18, 19]. As a traditional coalescent, ARC model assumes neutral evolution, constant population size with random mating and uniformity of recombination rates across the genome, as well as straightforward extension on complex demographic events. The key parameter in determining patterns of LD is the product of the per-generation recombination (c), and the effective population size (N_e): $\rho=4N_ec$, where ρ is the population recombination rate. Studies such as sperm typing or pedigree analysis, counting the recombination events in one generation, can be used to calculate c, which depends on genomic features such as local DNA motif; while ρ, which depends on demographic history (effect on N_e), and therefore differs substantially among populations.

The numerous methods and statistics based on ARC can be classified into summary statistics, full-likelihood approaches and approximate-likelihood approaches[20, 24]. Summary statistics, though very easy to calculate, provides limited information and is therefore rarely used at present. Full-likelihood approaches try to incorporate all information contained in the data and always integrate many variable dimension genealogies. In this way, Markov Chain Monte Carlo (MCMC), Bayesian MCMC and important sampling (IS) have been used to estimate the likelihood surface for model parameters[20, 25]. For examples, inspired by the observed patterns of recombination in sperm-typing studies, Wang and Rannala[24] developed a Bayesian full-likelihood method using MCMC to estimate background recombination rates and hotspots. However, it seems impossible to apply them on moderate dataset since they are notorious for computational intensity.

Up to now, various approximate-likelihood approaches have been developed to investigate the large population genetic data available[22, 26, 27]. However, these methods either ignore rare and low frequency genetic loci which harbor little information of recombination, or consider only a small number of sites at a time, calculating the likelihood of each subset separately and combining them to obtain the approximate likelihood. In the simplest case, maximum-likelihood estimator of the recombination parameter for each linked two-loci pair was calculated independently[27], and a composite-likelihood estimator was constructed by multiplying all pair-wise likelihood. This approach is not only able to handle both genotyping data and sequencing data efficiently, but also straightforward to incorporating complex mutation and population models with high accuracy. McVean *et al.*[22] extended the two-locus composite-likelihood approach by allowing different recombination rates between each pair of makers, and took a Bayesian implementation using prior distribution to avoid over-fitting, thus estimating recombination rates from a fine-scale of kilo-bases up to that of mega-bases.

Based on the observed ancestry switch points in admixed population, Hinch et al.[29] and Wegmann et al.[30] constructed a high-resolution recombination map of African American in 2000, respectively. It was novel to use ancestry-based approach to identify recombination events and recombination hotspots. Both studies showed that the recombination maps of admixed population are consistent with those of non-admixed populations at mega-bases levels. However, the recombination maps of the African American differ significantly from those of the European at fine-scale. In addition, Hinch *et al.*[29] also identified about 2,500 active recombination hotspots in African Americans but not in European. The 17bp DNA motif enriched in African specific hotspots is well matched to a predicted *PRDM9* binding alleles common in Africans. And individuals who carry the motif tend to have a higher risk of the disease-causing genomic rearrangements. Wegmann *et al.*[30] showed that recombination rates at regions with known large chromosomal structural variants, especially inversions, are likely to be highly population specific compared with those at other regions.

2.6 Inference of effective population size from genetic data

The effective population size (N_e) is defined as the number of breeding individuals in an idealized population that shows the same allele frequency spectrum as the population under consideration. N_e is an important parameter in population genetics that helps to explain population demographic history and genetic structure of complex traits. It is also an important parameter in conservation biology, ecology and evolutionary biology[31]. Based on heterozygosity, LD, temporal changed allele frequency and pattern of genetic variation within or between populations, various strategies and methods have been proposed to estimate current, past and ancient N_e[32].

In recent years, the most quickly developed methodology for estimating N_e was based on LD. Hayes *et al.*[33] proposed chromosome segment homozygosity (CSH), a new statistics, to estimate N_e in different time scales using haplotype or haplotype frequencies data. CSH is the probability of two homologous chromosomal segments coming from the same ancestor without recombination interference. When population size changes linearly over time, the expectation of CSH will be $1/(4N_tc + 1)$, where N_t is the effective population size at t=1/2c generations ago, and c is the length of the chromosome segment in morgans. Thus, CSHs for chromosomal segments of different length can be used to estimate the Ne at different time scales. In other words, CSH over a long distance reflects recent N_e, whereas that over a short distance reflects N_e far more back. When the statistics was applied on human haplotype data[33], N_e was estimated to be ~5,000 at about 2,000 generations ago, and ~15,000 at about 182 generations ago. The results reflect an exponential growth of human population in the past.

The distribution of the time since the most recent common ancestor (TMRCA) between two alleles cherishes much information about population demographic history[34]. In order to take advantage of the genome-wide sequencing data, Li and Durbin[34, 35] proposed a pairwise sequentially Markovian coalescent (PSMC) model that scaled mutation, recombination and piecewise ancestral population size to reveal the detailed population history. In the PSMC-HMM model[34], the observation is a binary sequence of '0', '1' and '.'. The emission probability from state t is $e(1|t) = e^{-\theta t}$, $e(0|t) = 1-e^{-\theta t}$, and $e(.|t) = 1$; the transition probability from s to t is:

$$p(t \mid s) = (1 - e^{-\rho t}) q(t \mid s) + e^{-\rho s} \delta(t - s)$$

where θ and ρ is the scaled mutation rate and recombination rate, respectively; $\delta(.)$ is the Dirac delta function and

$$q(t \mid s) = \frac{1}{\lambda(t)} \int_0^{\min\{s,t\}} \frac{1}{s} \times e^{-\int_u^t \frac{dv}{\lambda(v)}} du$$

is the transition probability condition on there being a recombination event, where $\lambda(t) = N_e(t)/N_0$ is the relative population size at t. Li and Durbin[34] applied the PSMC model on seven high accurate individual genomes from Africa, Europe and East Asia, whose results showed that all populations shared similar N_e between 150 and 1,500 thousand year (kyr) ago. The N_e of African is different from that of non-African populations around 100-120 kyr ago (at 110 kyr ago, N_e of African = 15,313 ± 559; N_e of non-African = 12,829 ± 485). The estimated N_e of European and East Asian populations before 11 kyr ago were almost the same as both experienced a serious bottleneck between 150 kyr and 20-40 kyr ago, during which time their N_e declined from 13,500 to 1,200, and increased sharply afterwards.

3. Human origins, population structure and population history

3.1 Human origins and its early history

Although population genetics focus on variation changes within species, emergence of new species due to long population divergence is also an interesting topic. Recent theoretical studies have focused on the "Isolation with Migration" model of population divergence, which integrated many parameters using methods of population genetics[36]. It is known that genus *Homo* diverged from Australopithecines about 2.3 to 2.5 million years ago in Africa[37]. However, no species except modern human (*Homo sapiens*) in the genus *Homo* has survived in the long evolutionary history. Traditionally, there are two major competing models on the origin of our anatomically modern human: Recent African origin and multiregional evolution. The debates focus on whether modern human originated solely in

Africa. The former proposes that all modern human originated in Africa and dispersed into other parts of the world; while the latter holds that local *archaic hominin* evolved into modern human separately. With evidences from both mtDNA and Y chromosome, recent African origin model has been widely accepted and become the mainstream since the end of last century[38-40]. According to this model, *archaic hominin* evolved into anatomically modern humans solely in Africa about 200,000 years ago. Then a branch of modern humans left Africa 125,000 to 60,000 years ago, and replaced earlier *archaic hominin* such as Neanderthals and *Homo erectus* in other parts of the world.

However, mtNDA or Y chromosome only represents a genetic locus and is suffered from serious genetic drift. Analyses of two extinct *archaic hominin* genomes have enriched our understanding of human origins[41, 42]. The first sequenced *archaic hominin* was Neanderthal, the closest evolutionary cousin of present modern human, who used to live in large parts of Western Eurasia before extinction 30,000 years ago. Analysis of Neanderthal genome essentially supported the recent African origin of modern human. However, Neanderthal shared more genetic variants with present modern humans in Eurasia than in sub-Saharan Africa, which suggested that gene flow from Neanderthals into the ancestry of non-African occurred before the divergence of Eurasian groups[41].It is estimated that 1%-4% of the DNA in modern Eurasia is contributed by Neanderthal. Another sequenced *archaic hominin* was referred to as 'Denisovans' due to their bones was found in Denisova Cave in southern Siberia, who shared a common origin with Neanderthals[42]. Denisovans was not involved in the putative gene flow from Neanderthals into Eurasians; however, data analysis suggested that it has contributed 4–6% of DNA to present Melanesian. Gene flows from Denisovans to New Guineans, Australians, and Mamanwa were also found, but not to mainland East Asians, western Indonesians, Jehai, and Onge[43].

In 2011, genome of an aboriginal Australian, whose DNA was extracted from a 100-year-old lock of hair, was sequenced[44]. Genomic evidences showed that aboriginal Australians were descendents of population colonizing Australian about 62,000 to 75,000 years ago, which is different from that of modern East Asians possibly 25,000 to 38,000 years ago. Thus, present aboriginal Australians should be descendents of the earliest Australian colonist, possibly representing one of the oldest continuous populations outside Africa. In a nutshell, recent studies based on genome-wide data essentially support that all modern human originated in Africa and dispersed into other parts of the world by at least two waves. However, gene flows from some archaic hominin contributed to the gene pool of modern non-African.

3.2 Inference of population history from allele frequency spectrum

Analysis of allele frequency spectrum is one of the most commonly used strategies to infer population history. For example, a large proportion of rare alleles indicates recent population expansion, as mutations occurred since population expansions do not have enough time to spread. Based on expected allele frequency spectrum, various methods, such as those provided by Nielson[45] and Williamson *et al.*[46], have been developed to infer the demographic history. Several studies used multiple summary statistics to compare empirical data with that of simulations under varying demographic history. For example, Voight *et al.*[47] used level of polymorphism, allele frequency spectrum and LD to fit population bottleneck of non-African population. After correcting the ascertainment in HapMap data, Keinan *et al.*[48] found that both ancestry of East Asian and that of European experienced population bottlenecks out of Africa, with the former being affected more seriously.

3.3 Population structure and human history

An ideal population is a single entity in which all members randomly mates. However, because of geographic barriers and limited tendency for individuals to spread, natural populations rarely interbreed as in theoretical model, which leads to population structure. Elucidating human population structure can not only improve our knowledge on human population history, but also reduce false-positive results caused by population stratification in association studies. The worldwide population samples were essential for studying the global pattern of human population structure. Promoted by Cavalli-Sforza et al. in the 1990s, the Human Genome Diversity Project (HGDP) provided more than 1000 samples in 53 indigenous populations from the world[49]. The traditional methods for studying population structure could be classified into phylogeography and summary statistics[50]. These methods analyzed the genetic variation based on predefined populations/ethnics classification according to culture or geographic locations, which may not reflect the true genetic relationships. The clustering methods such as STRUCTURE[51, 52] can infer the population genetic structure directly without the prior information about the origins of individuals. STRUCTURE implements a model-based clustering method that integrates Markov chain Monte Carlo (MCMC) to infer population structure with multi-locus genotype data. Rosenberg et al.[53] applied STRUCTURE on 1,056 HGDP individuals genotyping at 377 microsatellites and found that individuals from the same predefined populations always shared similar membership coefficient in inferred clusters. When the number of clusters was set to five, the genetic clusters correspond to the five geographic regions (Africa, East Asia, America, Oceania and Europe) very well [53]. In order to take advantage of the genome-wide high-density data, many computationally efficient software and algorithms have been developed[54, 55]. Based on a new method, it is found that seven genetic clusters correlate well with the seven major geographic regions, namely African, Middle East, Europe, Central/South Asia, East Asia, America and Oceania[56].

Multivariate techniques have been used to condense information of numerous loci into one or a few synthetic variables, which are especially powerful in analyzing the genome-wide high-density data. Principle component analysis (PCA) has been introduced to population genetics by Cavalli-Sforza and his colleagues[57] >30 years ago. Interests in PCA were renewed after Patterson *et al.*[58] had implemented it on individual genotypic data and plotted individuals on the graph. McVean[59] showed that for SNP data, the projection of samples onto the PCs could be obtained directly from the average coalescent times between pairs of haploid genomes. These results provided a framework for interpreting PCA projections in terms of underlying processes, including migration, geographical isolation, and admixture. McVean also demonstrated a link between PCA and Wright's F_{ST}[59]. Reich et al.[60] suggested that PCA was very useful in population genetics and highlighted three applications: detecting population substructure, correcting stratification in association studies and making qualified inferences about human history. For example, the first PC map based on European populations showed a southeast-to-northwest cline and was interpreted as the reflection of Neolithic farming spreading from the Levant to Europe about 6,000-9,000 years ago[57]. And the hypothesis about the expansion of Neolithic farming has been supported by many genetic and archaeological data[60, 61]. However, according to the study by Novembre and Stephens[62], PCs correlating with geography do not necessarily reflect major population migrations but isolation by distance, in which gene exchanges are only among neighboring populations. For example, based on the dataset of 3,000 individuals genotyped at over half a million SNPs, Novmbre et al.[63] found that the inferred principle components essentially reconstructed the geographic map of European, thus they suggested that individual genome could be used to infer the geographic origin of the individuals.

3.4 Integrating haplotype information to infer population relationships and history

Recently, methods and statistics that integrate LD and haplotype information to infer population relationships and history have been developed, which may become the mainstream of population genetics in the future. The studies integrating haplotype information essentially have greatly improved our knowledge on the human history and population relationships. For example, the LD information has been integrated into STRUCTURE as linkage model to estimate the ancestry along chromosome[51]. The average length of the migrant chromosome tracts were used to infer the change of recent gene flow in different populations[64]. In particular, based on a copying model adapted from Li and Stephens[65], the worldwide LD pattern of human was used to infer human origins and dispersals[66]. The study also found some new points on the human history such as the most northerly East-Asian population (Yakut) having received genetic contribution from the ancestors of north European. The copying model was further used to estimate parameters of population split, which illustrated LD pattern carrying historical information beyond recent migration[67].

Haplotype-sharing, which accounts for LD and haplotype information, has been proposed to infer the human history[68, 69]. For example, haplotype analysis has been used in the study on human genetic diversity in Asia[69]. With diversity decreasing from south to north, haplotype diversity was found strongly correlated with latitude (R^2 = 0.91, P < 0.0001), which was constant with a loss of diversity as populations moved to higher latitudes. Besides, more than 90% haplotypes in East Asian population could be found in Southeast and Central-South Asian populations, of which about 50% were found in Southeast only, and 5% in Central-South Asian only. Phylogenic analyses of private haplotypes indicate greater similarity between East Asian and Southeast Asian, suggesting that Southeast Asia was a major geographic source of East Asian population. Another example, although Uyghurs have been proposed as a genetic donor of the East Asian[66], haplotype-sharing analysis of Uyghur showed that more than 95% of Uyghur haplotype could be found in either European or East Asian population, which contradicts the expectation of null hypothesis. Simulation studies further indicated that the proportion of Uyghur private haplotype observed in the empirical data is only expected in alternative models assuming Uyghur is an admixed population[68].

Furthermore, Xu and Jin[12] proposed chromosome-wide haplotype sharing (CHS) as a measure of genetic similarity between human populations, which was an indirect approach to integrate recombination information. They showed that recombination and genetic differences between human populations are strongly correlated in both empirical and simulated data, indicating that recombination events in different human populations are evolutionarily related. They further demonstrated that CHS could be used to reconstruct reliable phylogenies of human populations and the majority of the variation in CHS matrix could be attributed to recombination[12]. However, for distantly related populations, the utility of CHS to reconstruct correct phylogeny is limited, suggesting that the linear correlation of CHS and population divergence could have been disturbed by recurrent recombination events over a large time scale. The CHS they proposed is a practical approach without involving computationally challenging and time-consuming estimation of recombination parameter. The advantage of CHS is rooted in its integration of both drift and recombination information, thus providing additional resolution especially for populations separated recently.

4. Natural selection and human adaptation to local environments

4.1 Genome-wide detection of natural selection

One of the most exciting prospects of genome-wide high-density polymorphic data is its implication in detecting natural section. Before the advent of genomic era, detecting natural selection was exclusively through candidate gene studies, in which a gene was priori hypothesized subjected to natural selection and the value of statistic on it was compared with that under neutrality[70]. However, besides the inefficiency, there are three significant limitations of candidate gene studies. Firstly, a priori hypothesis under which gene has been subjected to natural selection requires priori understanding of the gene functions or genotype-phenotype relationships. Genetic basis for most traits/phenotypes remaining mysterious limited our ability to intelligently nominate candidate genes for investigation[71]. Secondly, since demographic events such as population expansion can leave footprints on the genome similar to that of natural selection, the statistical power of candidate study for identifying genes under natural selection is confounded[72]. Thirdly, candidate gene study is especially inefficient in detecting selection in regulatory elements that are far from coding regions.

The availability of genomic data has offered a new paradigm for detecting signature of natural selection, which was referred to as genomic approach. In addition to the high throughput, it also shows several statistical advantages[70, 71]. First, it searches the whole genome without a priori hypothesis which gene is under selection, yielding a set of unbiased results. Second, since demographic history affects genomic loci equally while natural selection only affect a few loci, it provides a framework to distinguish natural selection signals from demographic history in principle. Third, genomic approach does not need a priori knowledge about the gene functions and genotype-phenotype relationships. With all these being said, genomic approach is extremely efficient and powerful compared with the traditional candidate approach. The most commonly used genomic approach is the "outlier of summary statistic"[71], in which a large number of sites are examined, calculating a statistic across all loci that quantifies a specific features of genetic variations, constructing empirical distribution, and defining selection candidate based on the extreme tail of the empirical distribution. Although simulations under neutrality have been conducted either to guide the definition of thresholds or to evaluate the efficiency of the outlier method, criteria for defining outlier in most studies is often arbitrary, e.g., loci falling in 99th percentile of the empirical distribution[71].

Up to now, hundreds of genome-wide studies have been conducted to detect natural selection in human, and the initial maps of positive selection in human have been produced.

Although these maps are incomplete, error-prone, and of low-resolution, it is no doubt that this progress has fundamentally changed the field of human population genetics and evolutionary studies.

4.2 Genetic basis and statistics for detecting selection using genome-wide data

As we know, selective sweep acts on the beneficial allele and makes its frequency increase quickly, and ultimately affects a large region around it due to LD. Therefore, the features of genetic variation subjected to natural selection in a region would be different from those evolve neutrally. Various methods have been developed, taking advantage of the footprints left by selection, such as changed allele frequency spectrum, increased derived allele frequencies, polymorphism deviating from interspecies divergence, population differentiation and exteneded haplotype homozygosity. However, we only introduce the recently developed methods and those whose statistical power greatly benefit from the genome-wide high-density data.

1. Extended haplotype homozygosity (EHH)

Under neutral model, it takes a long time for a new mutation to drift to high frequency in a population, during which time LD around this variant will decay substantially due to recombination[73, 74]. However, positive selection leads to rapid increase of the frequency of beneficial allele, occurring in such a short time that recombination does not have time to break the selected haplotype. Thus, an allele having extremely long LD compared with its counterparts should be seen as a signal of recent positive selection. Based on this principle, many different statistics such as EHH and integrated haplotype score (iHS) were developed[74-77]. EHH[74] is defined as the probability that two randomly chosen chromosomes carrying a tested core haplotype are homozygous at all SNPs. While iHS compares the EHH decay around an ancestral and derived allele[76]. Compared with other approaches, the most obvious advantage of these approaches is that they are relatively robust in choosing genetic markers or ascertainment bias[74]. Although it is pretty powerful to detect recent positive selection, it has little power in revealing natural selection happened about tens of thousands of years ago, because most chromosomal segments will be split into small pieces less than 100kb by recombination after 30, 000 years.

2. Population differentiation

Population differentiation is largely determined by population demographic history and genetic drift[78], which almost affect each locus similarly. However, variations of local environment impose different selection pressures on some genomic regions, leading to high population differentiation at these regions[79]. The first genome-wide study on positive selection taking advantage of population differentiation was based on the locus-specific F_{ST}[79]. Compared with others, this method is much more powerful in detecting ancient selective sweep that happened tens of thousands of years ago[80]. Another strategy based on population differentiation was the cross-population extended haplotype homozygosity (XP-EHH)[77], which is much powerful in detecting recent selection less than 1,000 generations. Recently, Chen *et al.*[81] developed a new method for detecting selective sweeps that involves jointly modeling the multi-locus allele frequency differentiation between two populations.

These methods were much robust to both ascertainment bias and recombination rate heterogeneity. However, these approaches cannot be directly applied on recently admixed population due to the confused population structure. Jin et al.[82] developed a new strategy to detect natural selection in admixed population such as African American, in which they reconstructed an ancestral African population (AAF) from African components of ancestry in African American and compared the population differentiation between indigenous African and AAF. Many targets of selection identified by this approach were associated with African-Americans specific high-risk diseases such as prostate cancer and hypertension, suggesting an important role these disease-related genes might have played in adapting to new environments[82].

3. Biased ancestry contribution in admixed populations

Under neutral evolution, the locus-specific ancestral contribution for all loci were similar, if not equal, as genetic drift on all loci were simultaneous[83]. However, a beneficial allele from an ancestry may provide higher survival or reproduction capability for the admixed individuals, leading to the increase of ancestral contribution from population carrying the beneficial allele. Thus, some genomic regions in admixed population might show excess of a particular ancestry, possibly attributable to selection pressures after the population admixture[84]. By far, several studies have used the genome-wide data to scan for signatures of selection in admixed populations[82].

4. Composite strategies and new challenge

Although hundreds of regions subjected to positive selection have been identified, most of the underlying genes and causal mutations are still unknown. A recent study by Grossman *et al.*[85] analyzed five statistics (F_{ST}, XP-EHH, iHS, ΔiHH, ΔDAF) and found their values were highly correlated only around the causal variants. Based on this observation, composite of multiple signals (CMS), a composite likelihood test, was proposed to distinguish causal variants. For each statistic *i*, the probability *P* of a score s_i was estimated whether selected or not. Assuming a uniform prior probability of selection π, the CMS score is the approximate posterior probability that the variant is selected:

$$CMS = \prod_{i=1}^{n} \frac{P(s_i \mid selected) \times \pi}{P(s_i \mid selected) \times \pi + P(s_i \mid unselected) \times (1-\pi)}$$

Application of CMS to HapMap data has localized population-specific selective signals to 55kb, and identified known or novel causal variants[85]. It is novel to use composite strategy to identify causal variants, although several studies have proposed statistics considering multiple factors or combining several summary statistics.

Most aforementioned statistics and strategies detecting natural selection were developed according to the classic selective model in which a new beneficial mutation arises and increases in frequency to fix in a population[70, 71]. However, using the 1000 Genome Project data, Hernandez *et al.*[86] showed that classic selective sweeps were rare in recent human evolution, which indicates that many statistics may loose power in detecting selections that have not been modeled and considered. Thus it is a big challenge to depict, model and detect the signatures of natural selection in recent human evolutionary history.

4.3 Human adaptation to local environments

There are many completely distinguished environments on the earth, varying in temperature, moisture, light, and so on. Most animals and plants can only survive in a specific environment, even chimpanzee, our closest relative, has very limited distribution in Africa. Modern human, however, have successively colonized almost every corner of the earth within only about 100,000 years since the first branch of modern human left Africa[87]. Although the current patterns of human genetic and phenotypic diversities can, to some extent, be explained by human migration and demographic history[56], natural selection and adaptive evolution have also played very important roles in different populations adapting to local environments, as revealed by modern genetics[77, 88].

Natural selection acts on the phenotypes only when their differentiations correspond with different survival or reproductive rates, which makes the advantageous phenotypes and their underlying genetic variants become more common in a population. Over time, this process results in adaptive evolution, allowing organisms to handle the challenges from the environment to ensure their survival and reproduction. For example, animal is initially able to accommodate to the environmental challenges by simply changing their behaviors such as daily activities, and if the behavioral flexibility does not work, a range of physiological mechanisms accompanied by regulations of gene expression, such as accumulation of body fat, will act to relieve the environmental pressures. However, if the aforementioned mechanisms fail to buffer against the environmental challenges, the survival and reproductive rates began to vary from individual to individual. In this case, individuals harboring advantageous allele are more likely to have higher survival rates or have more descendents, thus frequencies of the advantage alleles increased accordingly, giving an indication of natural selection and adaptive evolution.

As a key mechanism of modern evolution, natural selection, supported by various scientific evidences, has been widely accepted at present. Although our species was not discussed in *On the Origin of Species* published in 1859 considering the religious Europe, the theory of evolution has gradually been applied to understanding human variation in the following years. Identifying targets of positive selection in human based on candidate gene studies has been frustratingly slow for just a decade. Recently, with the availability of large-scale genotyping and sequence data, we have experienced an explosive increase of studies on genome-wide scanning for signals of selection[71, 89]. Identification of genomic regions showing evidence of natural selection has helped us to find genes adapting populations to pathogens, climate, diet and possible cognitive challenges. These discoveries have greatly enriched our understanding of human origins and history, and hold large potential for identifying genes with important biological functions, thus in turn, will elucidate the genetic basis of some human diseases[71, 77]. These studies together provide many new insights into the natural selection process and mechanisms, which will ultimately improve the modern evolution theory.

4.4 Human adaptation to high-latitude climates

The early migration out of Africa exposed ancestral populations to colder environments with less sunlight, which eventually left the most obvious footprints on human populations[90]. Human morphology such as body mass, body mass index (BMI), nasal size, hair texture and density, lip size and thinness, relative sitting height (RSH) and surface area/body mass ratio have been reported shaped by climate adaptation[91]. Among all these characteristics, skin pigmentation is perhaps the most conspicuous one, with darker-skinned populations concentrated in the tropics, and lighter-skinned populations in higher latitudes[92, 93]. In fact, skin pigmentation is primarily determined by the type, amount and distribution of melanin. The global distribution of melanin can be explained by the balance selections interacting between elusion of ultraviolet radiation and photosynthesis of vitamin D_3[92, 93]. In tropic regions, the dark melanin protects people from sunburn by scattering and absorbing ultraviolet radiation, as well as limiting photo-degradation of nutrients such as folate. In this case, any mutation that impacts normal dark melanin production is deleterious, therefore, genes involved in dark melanin production such as *MC1R* are subjected to strong purifying selection in African[94]. Contrarily, the situation is very different for non-African including European, East Asian, and Southeast Asian, where *MC1R* is highly polymorphic, containing many nonsynonymous variants. In higher latitude, with less sunlight available, depigmentation may be favored since ultraviolet penetration is necessary for vitamin D_3 synthesis. Therefore, those genes that are associated with light skin such as *SLC45A2* and *OCA2* have been subjected to recent positive selection[95]. In order to cope with the ultraviolet radiation in temperate zone, human have developed a complex tanning system that includes immediate pigment darkening and delayed tanning reaction.

Although polymorphisms in *ASIP* and *OCA2* may play a shared role in shaping light skin around the world[95], it seems that the evolutions of light skin color in East Asia and western Eurasia are independent of each other, with many different genes underlying the environmental adaptation[77, 88, 95]. Based on extended haplotype homozygosity (EHH) or extremely high population differentiation using high density SNPs data, it is revealed that *SLC45A2* and *SLC24A5* have been subjected to strong positive selection in western Eurasia, while *EADR* and *ED2R* in East Asia and America[77]. Especially, the global distributions of both *CLC24A5* A111T polymorphism and *EDAR* V370A polymorphism correlate very well with the ethnic skin characteristics.

After long evolution since human out of Africa, the general populations have adapted to local environments to some extent. However, due to recent human migrations and colonization, many people lived in geographic region with completely different environmental conditions compared with their ancestry, which led to many health problems. For examples, fair skinned individuals living in low latitude are at much higher risk of skin cancer, while dark skinned individuals living in high latitude are at higher risk of vitamin D deficiency. Especially, European Australian are at about 10 times higher risk of several types of skin cancers than Australian aboriginals[92], while African American have the highest risk of vitamin D deficiency[96].

Meanwhile, our ancestry in tropic Africa also evolved a series of mechanisms to accommodate to the local environment (heat-adaptation), which include cooling through sweating[90]. As we know, sweating is accompanied by salt loss at the same time. Therefore, the low dietary salt in local environment ultimately leads to the selection for salt retention. After blood volume was depleted as a result of water loss, individuals with stronger arterial tone and cardiac contractile force are more likely to survive. However, this advantage may turn out to be negative when population migrated to temperate climate and will ultimately lead to hypertension. This has been supported by the genetic evidences from worldwide populations, including the functional alleles of seven genes, which are associated with distribution of blood pressure showing a latitudinal cline[97]. It is shown that *GNB3* 825T (one allele) accounts for a remarkable 64% of worldwide variation in blood pressure. Peoples from tropic climate migrating to temperate climate recently show high susceptibility to hypertension, which is represented by African-Americans[98, 99].

4.5 Human adaptation to high-altitude

Although latitude cline is the main pattern of human phenotype variations, another impressive example is the high-altitude adaptation. The environmental challenges for human survival and reproduction in high altitude include deceased ambient oxygen tension, increased ultraviolet radiation, extreme diurnal ranging in temperature, arid climate and so on. In particular, high-altitude hypoxia, caused by the decreased barometric pressure in high altitude, cannot be overcome simply by behavioral and cultural modification. However, there are approximately 140 million individuals living permanently at high-altitude (above 2500 meters) in North, Central and South America, East Africa, and Asia[100, 101]. Populations living at the high altitude, especially those living at Tibetan Plateau and Andes, have evolved unique physiological characteristics compared with each other and with low altitude populations[102]. It is known that Andean population, as well as high altitude sojourners, demonstrated higher hemoglobin concentration than low-altitude populations. In contrast, Tibetan populations exhibit lower hemoglobin concentrations than expected[102]. The physiological characteristics of the high altitude residents also include blunted ventilatory response to acute hypoxia, protection from altitude-associated fetal growth restriction and so on[100, 103].

Although the physiology of these populations has been well described for hundreds of years, the genetic basis of these traits has not been revealed until recently. Several studies, using different technologies and strategies, have identified the genes that adapted Tibetans to the local environment based on genome-wide data[80, 101, 104, 105]. The candidate genes identified by these studies are essentially consistent with each other. The strongest ones are *EGLN1* (also known as *HIFPH2*, located in 1q42.2) and *EPAS1* (also known as *HIF2A*, located in 2p21), both of which are involved in HIF pathway and response to hypoxia[80, 104, 105]. Xu *et al.*[80] analyzed the local linkage disequilibrium (LD) of the two HIF genes and ultimately found the Tibetans dominant haplotype. Based on the significant overrepresentation of the carrier of dominant haplotype of *EPAS1* and *EGLN1* in Tibetans, they proposed a "dominant haplotype carrier" model to explain the roles of the two genes in adapting to high altitude[80].

4.6 Human adaptation to shifted diet

Diet is one of the most important factors in species evolution and has been highlighted in *On the Origin of Species*. Our ancestry had adapted their genome to the food from local environment in evolutionary history. However, facilitated by the development of stone tools, the master of fire and the recent domestication of plants and animals[106, 107], human evolution is characterized by significant dietary shifts. Especially, the diet and lifestyle conditions have been changed fundamentally since the introduction of agriculture and the industrial revolution. The conflicts between the genetically determined biological features and contemporary diet and lifestyle may lead to the diseases of civilization[108]. A common view is that post-Neolithic human adapted, through a 'thrifty genotypes', to a hunter-gather lifestyle of feast and famine[109, 110]. However, studies based on the recent available genome-wide data showed that the real case might be complex[111].

Lactase persistence of human is one of the best-studied examples of dietary adaptation. Lactase-phlorizin hydrolase (*LPH*) is predominantly expressed in small intestine, where it hydrolyzes lactose into glucose and galactose that can be easily absorbed[112]. In human, the capability to digest lactose, the main carbohydrate in milk, declines rapidly after weaning because of the decreasing levels of *LPH*. However, using lactose as a source of food and nutrient in adulthood provides some survival advantages for populations mainly on dairy food. It is found that distribution of lactase persistence correlates well with that of populations with a history of cattle domestication and milk drinking[113]. The lactase persistence is inherited as a dominant mendelian trait, and is thought caused by change of *cis*-acting element of *LCT*, the gene encoding LPH[114]. A linkage disequilibrium (LD) and haplotype analysis of Finnish pedigrees has identified a causative regulatory variant (C/T-13910) ~14kb upstream of *LCT* gene[112], with an estimated age of about 2,000-20,000 years[115]. A region of extensive LD spanning >1M has been observed in European chromosome with T-13910 allele, which is consistent with recent positive selection[10, 115, 116]. However, lactase persistent populations elsewhere such as African do not carry this variant[117]. Association studies on Tanzanians, Kenyans and Sudanese identified another three variants (G/C-14010, T/G-13915 and C/G-13907) that could lead to lactase persistence. These SNPs originated on different haplotype backgrounds from European C/T-13910 and from each other, which indicated the independent origin of lactase persistence[117]. Genotyping across a 3-Mb region demonstrated haplotype homozygosity extending >2Mb in chromosomes carrying C-14010, which is consistent with a selective sweep about 7,000 years ago. The different origins of lactase persistence also provide a perfect example of convergent evolution due to strong selective pressure as the shared dietary culture.

However, starch consumption is the prominent characteristic of agricultural societies, especially among the populations living on planting. Interestingly, *AMY1* (human salivary amylase gene) has been reported subjected to recent positive selection in populations with planting tradition, contrasting to *LCT* in population with stockbreeding tradition[106, 117], which might reflect the influence of different kinds of agricultures and cultures. Copy number of the salivary amylase gene (*AMY1*) are corrected positively with salivary amylase protein level and individuals from population with high-starch diets[106]. Thus individual with more copies of *AMY1* is presumably able to get more out of their starchy diet, thus providing survival advantage when food is limited. It is also suggested that higher *AMY1* copy number and protein levels might also buffer against the fitness-reducing effects of intestinal disease[106].

4.7 Adaptation to pathogens and its influence on defense genes

Infectious diseases have always been a massive burden in human evolutionary history. The human life expectancy was <25 years until the control of infections by improved hygiene, vaccines and antibiotics following the advent of Pasteur's microbial theory of disease[118]. Being a major cause of human mortality, pathogens also imposed strong selective pressure on the human genome. However, the relationship between pathogens and natural selection had not been established in a long time span, until John B. S. Haldane found the link by analyzing thalassaemia patients infecting malaria[119], one of the best examples showing how infectious disease shapes human genome and how natural selection is working. The pathogen adaptation process is more complex than any of the other kind of selection pressure as the evolutionary dynamics of host-pathogen interactions lead to constant selection for adaptation and counter-adaptation in the competing species. Through the contending with pathogens, human have to improve their immune defense mechanism to combat microbial infection.

Although human and chimpanzee split only about 3 million years ago, prevalence and severity of infectious disease such as HIV, *Plasmodium malaria*, hepatitis B, hepatitis C and influenza A between humans and non-human primates are different[120, 121]. In human populations, many genes involving in infectious diseases have also been revealed subjected to natural selection. Especially, many studies have demonstrated the correlation between genetics variability in human population worldwide and pathogen richness in the corresponding geographic regions[122, 123]. Genome-wide scans for positive selection have detected >5,000 genomic regions that present at least one genomic signals of positive selection[124]. When we focused on natural selection that occurred more recently (detected by integrated haplotype score and LD decay test), defense genes were found over-represented[76, 125]. These observations may indicate that our immune system has particularly been challenged during the recent phases of human evolution, which might propose a strong burden of infectious disease that are associated with the advent of agriculture at the beginning of the Neolithic period 10,000 years ago[126]. In this situation, genome-wide association studies (GWAS) has become a powerful tool in detecting loci associated with the susceptibility or severity of infectious diseases. These susceptibility genes identified in this way are targets, transports or some other components in the pathogen infectious pathway. Thus, careful analysis of the pathogens associated genes will finally illuminate the infectious process and the targets of selection.

The model in which human adapts to pathogens is very complex and dependents on a lot of factors, including the type of microorganism, the different temporal and spatial presence of pathogens during evolution, their varying pathogenicity, the nature of the host-pathogen interaction, and the rate at which pathogens evolve[124]. A study on Toll-like receptor (*TLR*) gene family has concluded that viruses have exerted stronger selective pressures than other pathogens by constraining amino acid diversity at viral recognition TLRs[127]. Although the immune-related genes played a role in protecting the host from infection, mutations that inactivate these genes are likely to represent a selective advantage for the host when a pathogen uses the host's immune receptors as a mechanism of cell entry and survival. Some of these genes have lost their function because of the strong selection pressure, which also provides insights into the degree of redundancy in our immune system[128]. Loss-of-function mutations in *CCR5*, *DARC*, *CASP12*, *SERPINA2* and *SIGLEC12* are such examples. However, the selection may be very complex sometimes considering the changing pathogens. For example, CCR5-Δ32 allele is a deletion mutation of *CCR5* gene that impairs the function of its coding protein and has a specific impact on the function of T cells. It has been subjected to positive selection in Europe and can block the entrance of HIV-1[129]. However, since HIV has not emerged in Europe until recently, the selection signals on *CCR5*-Δ32 might be caused by Black Death or/and smallpox[130]

There are many well-studied examples about the natural selection imposed by pathogens, among which the selection imposed by malaria may be the best. Malaria has been, and still is, one of the major causes of child mortality in tropical regions[131]. Because of the strong selective pressure, malaria has become the driven force of most common Mendelian diseases including sickle-cell anemia, α-thalassemia, β-thalassemia, glucose-6-phosphatase (*G6PD*) deficiency and so on. However, these erythrocyte variants are probably only the tip of the iceberg considering all the genes associated with susceptibility and resistance to malaria, many of which are involved in immune system and inflammatory genes[132]. All these evidences suggested that malaria was the strongest known force of evolution in recent human history. The observations that different malaria-resistance alleles arose in different regions suggested independent evolutionary history of these genes[132].

5. Complex diseases/traits: Genetic basis and identification of the underlying variants

5.1 Overview of complex diseases/traits

Complex traits (or multifactorial traits) refer to phenotypes that vary in degree and can be attributed to the effects of multiple genes in combination with environmental factors. Generally, complex traits contribute to what we see as continuous characteristics in organisms, such as height, skin color, and body mass, whose inheritances do not follow Mendel's law. Most human diseases, such as diabetes, hypertension and various cancers, can be thought as some special complex traits, and are also associated with multiple genes and environmental factors. In fact, most studies only focus on the complex diseases due to their great health implications. Current debates concerning the genetic basis of complex diseases focus on two hypotheses: Common disease common variants (CDCV) and common disease rare variants (CDRV)[133, 134]. The CDCV hypothesis argues that the major genetic susceptibility to the complex/common disease are variations with appreciable frequency in the population, but relatively low penetrance[135, 136], while the alternative CDRV hypothesis argues that multiple rare variations with high penetrance are the major contributors[137, 138].

Technology advance on DNA microarray has lured many scientists genotyping high-density SNPs on thousands of individuals. Up to now, GWAS have reproducibly identified thousands of genes associated with complex diseases/traits[139, 140], providing many new insights into the functional and biological networks of these genes. However, among these heritable components of complex disease, only a small fraction has been explained. A potential source of the majority of missing heritability is the contribution of rare variants. Although next generation sequencing has the potential to discover the entire spectrum of sequence variation in well-phenotyped individuals, it remains a challenge to develop efficient methods to integrate the rare variants and eliminate the effects of sequence error and missing data.

5.2 Models for allelic spectrum of complex diseases

Allelic spectrum is the total variations that contribute to a disease, including common variants (frequency >1%), rare variants (frequency <1%), high penetrance and low penetrance. The allelic spectrum of complex disease has important influence on both research and clinical practice. In brief, it determines the strategies and methodologies for disease gene discovery. Although various methods and statistics have been developed by simply assuming high or intermediate allele frequency, allelic spectrums of the discovered susceptibility are seemingly to be complex. Since human population experienced complicated demographic history and a series of local adaptations, it is still obscure how human history affects the allelic spectrum of complex disease.

Despite the fact that several studies have promoted the formulation of the common disease common variants (CDCV) hypothesis, it turns out to be a complete hypothesis after the publication of the allelic spectrum of human disease by Reich and Lander[141], in which they used empirical data to qualify the allelic spectrum of rare diseases and studied the changes of allele frequency under rapid population expansion. As a result, they found that CDCV is not incompatible with the reported susceptible variants and diseases. They predicted that the overall frequencies of disease alleles are not low and it is possible to use variants with allele frequency above a threshold to detect the susceptible loci. The ancestral-susceptibility model provides an evolutionary framework to explain the susceptibility alleles to be ancestral alleles (mostly common alleles)[135]. According to this model, the ancestral alleles reflect ancient human populations adaptation, whereas the derived alleles were deleterious. However, with the shift of environment and lifestyle, the ancestral alleles increase the risk of common diseases in modern populations.

Many studies have challenged CDCV hypothesis and supported the alternative hypothesis common disease rare variants (CDRV). For example, Pritchard[137] argued that population processes such as mutation, genetic drift and purifying selection are against the deleterious alleles, which reduce the frequency of disease causal alleles. In this context, common variants, with an appreciable frequency, tend to be older and are unlikely to be subjected to long-lasting purifying selection in the whole evolutionary history. However, rare variants are either new mutations or being selected against owing to their deleterious nature. Furthermore, studies have found individuals with extreme values of quantitative phenotypes significantly cherished more rare missenses variants in candidate genes and pathways[138]. The evolutionary explanation for CDRV hypothesis is selection-mutation balance model, in which most missense mutations are deleterious[142].

Based on previous observations, a decanalization model was proposed to explain the origin of complex diseases[143]. It is known that stabilizing selection drives species to an optimum that takes an intermediate value among all possible values of phenotype. In the case of complex diseases, canalized traits will influence fewer individuals than those that lack a mechanism to reduce susceptibility. Importantly, persistent stabilizing selection not only removes the risk allele, but also reduces the additive genetic effects of alleles that are present in the gene pool or arisen by mutations[144]. In decanalization model, increased variants broaden the normal distribution, which leads to some individuals excess liability threshold, rather than horizontal shift of entire distribution. Since changes of epistasis interaction must have happened in decanalized case, it is expected to observe interactions among risk alleles. As risk alleles are not selected against in normal individuals, the canalized system can facilitate genetic drift. Therefore, the risk alleles underlying complex disease may be very similar to the normal allele frequency spectrum, and gene-gene interaction and genetic pathway must be considered in the identification of risk allele.

In fact, there are supporting evidences for each of these hypotheses[133, 142, 143, 145]. Although there may be some artifacts and most causal alleles are unknown[146], hundreds of GWAS have identified thousands of high frequency susceptible alleles[139], indicating that CDCV does have its place. As for CDRV, rare mutations in *ANGPTL4* caused reduce of triglycerides[147], while rare independent mutations in renal salt handling genes (*SLC12A3*, *SLC12A1* and *KCNJ1*) contributed to blood pressure[148]. Since next generation sequencing has become affordable recently, reports on rare variants are accumulated quickly. Type 2 diabetes (T2D), immune disorders and psychological disorders have been used as examples of decanalization model[143].

5.3 Genome-wide association studies (GWAS)

The availability of high-throughput genotyping technologies, as well as the major efforts to identify genome-wide genetic diversity, has made the genome-wide association studies (GWAS) become possible. Especially, HapMap provided nearly 4 million SNPs and characterized the genome-wide LD pattern and haplotype map[9, 10]. The debates on marker selection that determines the genomic coverage at early stage have boiled down to choose a limited range of commodity chips. Although higher density will increase genomic coverage, it does not equate increasing much power in most cases. With limited funding, the overall power might be maximized by genotyping more samples using less dense and less costly array[149]. Hundreds of genome-wide association studies (GWAS) have been conducted to identify common variations that are statistically associated with particular diseases[9, 139]. The first wave of large-scale GWAS has improved our knowledge on genetic basis of many complex traits/diseases[150]. For example, we have witnessed rapid expansion in numbers of susceptible loci for some diseases/traits, such as type 1 diabetes, type 2 diabetes, prostate cancer, inflammatory bowel disease, breast cancer, height, fat mass and lipid[139, 149]. These findings have provided many valuable clues to the allelic architecture of complex traits.

Most GWAS have featured case-control designs, which has raised issues about the selection of suitable cases and controls. Optimal selection of both cases and controls is important due to the fact that they will seriously affect statistical power of GWAS. Case selection has mainly focused on improvement of statistical power by enriching specific disease-predisposing alleles including minimizing phenotypic heterogeneity. Optimal selection of control samples remains more controversial, although the accumulating empirical data indicate that many commonly expressed concerns have been overstated[149]. One economic approach is to use common-control to study a series of diseases/traits such as what Wellcome Trust Case Control Consortium (WTCCC) has done[150]. Another more economic strategy is to use the genetic matched controls in public available control resources such as Illumina iControlDB (www.illumina.com). As for the sample size, the consensus view is clear: the more the better. Increasingly, GWAS are being extended from case-control designs to population-based cohorts which offer longitudinal measures of a wide range of quantitative traits and integrate the environmental factors for systematic analysis[149].

Another potential challenge for GWAS are the presence of undetected population stratification that can mimic the signals of association, thus leading to false positive and missing statistical power[151-153]. Although the influence of population structure caused by continental differentiation is serious, these outliers can be easily removed[150]. Therefore, the residual work on population substructure should focus on identifying the cryptic population stratification in a region or an ethnic group. As for the population stratification in European such as the north-south cline, differences between Jewish and non-Jewish have been revealed[154, 155]. Even in one single ethnic population such as Han Chinese, the obvious population stratification such as north-south cline is observed[156, 157]. Several methods and statistics have been developed to detect and adjust the population stratifications, even for continental structure such as African American[151, 158].

Conclusively, GWAS are a very powerful tool in investigating the genetic basis of complex diseases/traits. It is undoubtedly that it represents an important advance compared with 'candidate gene' studies in which limited variants and samples yielded many non-replicated results. Based on a threshold of p-values $< 1.0 \times 10^{-5}$ and studies with >100,000 SNPs in the initial stage, overall 5,053 SNPs have been reported to be associated with hundreds of complex traits by September 24, 2011 (www.genome.gov) [139]. The deluge of GWAS also provided the opportunity to evaluate the potential impact of genetic variants on complex diseases by systematically cataloging and summarizing the characteristics of the identified trait/disease associated SNPs (TASs). Unsurprisingly, since GWAS were primarily powered for common variants, risk allele frequencies were well above 5% (interquartile range 21%-53%) in the populations analyzed as well as in the HapMap populations (CEU: 21-54%; YRI: 13-65%; CHB+JPT:13-58%)[139]. Based on the position and function of 465 unique TASs, 43% SNPs were located in intergenic regions, 45% were intronic, 9% were nonsynonymous, 2% were in 5'UTR or 3'UTR, and 2% were synonymous[139]. The odds ratios (ORs) of discrete traits ranged from 1.04 to 29.4 (median 1.33, interquartile range 1.20 –1.61). Evolutionary analysis of the diseases associated genes showed they have been subjected to stronger positive selection compared with that of background[159].

Although GWAS are a great success, most of the variants having been identified so far only account for a small increment in risk and explain a small fraction of estimated heritability. For example, human height is a classic complex traits with an estimated heritability of about 80%, however, with tens of thousands of individuals having been studied, more than 40 associated loci identified by GWAS explain only about 5% of phenotypic variance [160]. These phenomena have led to the heated discussion on where the missing heritability of the complex disease can be found[161]. Many explanations have been proposed, including much more variants of smaller effect that have not been identified, that rare variants are not examined in the commercial chips, epistasis undetected, epigenetic and structural variants poorly captured. From this point of view, GWAS are just a beginning in systematically identifying the disease-associated loci.

5.4 Association studies for next generation sequencing

Next-generation sequencing has the potential to discover the entire spectrum of sequence variations and has been proved to be successful in the study of Mendelian disorders[162, 163]. When association studies on expression quantitative trait loci (eQTL) were conducted using all SNPs in low-coverage pilot of the 1000 genome project, a large number of more significant eQTLs was observed compared with traditional chips[5]. Thus it is no doubt that next generation sequencing will greatly benefit the studies of complex traits/diseases in the future. However, the applications of it on complex disease studies, which generally require sequencing hundreds or thousands of individuals, remain to be a challenge due to the high costs and limits of sequencing capacity.

In order to take advantage of the next generation sequencing, three strategies have been proposed: imputation, genotyping and low-coverage sequencing[5, 163]. First, imputation of previously genotyped samples using the recent sequenced reference panel is the most economic way, albeit less accurate. Analysis of ~400 samples imputed based on 1000 genome project data has revealed that the imputed data have more power than the original genotyped data[5]. Second, commercial chips integrating the new discovered SNPs will essentially improve the statistical power in identifying the disease-associated sites. Third, low-coverage sequencing of many individuals can be used to detect polymorphic sites and infer genotypes when many individuals are sequenced (2-6 x coverage)[163]. However, low-coverage data include very high sequencing error and missing data compared with high-coverage data, which is a big challenge for genetic variants discovery and statistics of association study.

Since next generation sequence detects millions of rare variants, these data have three features: high proportion of rare variants, high error and high missing data[134]. Thus traditional statistics, testing the association of common alleles one by one, are not suitable for large amount of allelic heterogeneity presenting in sequencing data[164]. In recent years, various statistics have been proposed to analysis the coming data with new features[134, 165-167]. For examples, Li and Leal[165] developed a combined multivariate and collapsing (CMC) method taking advantage of both collapsing and multiple-marker tests, and demonstrated that CMC was both powerful and robust using sequencing data. Price et al.[167] proposed a method for detecting association of multiple rare variants based on regression of phenotypic values on individuals' genotype scores, integrating computational predications of the functional influences of missenses. Luo et al.[134] used a genome continuum model and functional principal components as a general principle to develop functional principal component analysis (FPCA) statistic for sequencing data.

5.5 Admixed population and admixture mapping

Strictly speaking, almost all human populations showed some admixture features to some extent. However, we usually only refer to the populations with recent ancestry from two or more continents as admixed populations, most of which arise from the colonization of America and trans-Atlantic slave trade. A substantial proportion of the populations in the New World are recent admixed populations, such as African Americans, Mestizos, Puerto Ricans and other Latino/Hispanic populations. In fact, admixed population also distributed in other parts of the world, such as Uyghur in Central Asia[68, 168, 169], and populations that are of African-Indian origin in South Asia[170, 171]. Although genetic differences between populations only represent a small fraction of the total genetic variation, some diseases have different prevalence in populations owing to local adaptation or genetic drift[172, 173]. In admixed population, high population differentiation allele between parental populations may be risk for a disease with varying prevalence. Therefore, local ancestry differentiation can be used for disease gene discovery, namely admixture mapping[174].

The statistical power of admixture mapping comes from the fact that population admixture creates LD between loci with different allele frequencies in ancestral parental populations[174-176]. Since population admixture creates extended LD and chromosomal segments of distinct ancestry even extending several cMs in recent admixed population, only thousands of (about 1,500-5,000) high ancestry informative markers (AIMs) will be enough for a genome-wide admixture mapping[177]. Factors influencing the statistical power of admixture mapping, such as admixture dynamics and demographic history, have been investigated in various studies[172, 176, 178, 179]. Admixture mapping using AIMs is very important for holding the statistical power and reducing costs[180]. As a kind of specialized GWAS, design of admixture mapping can be either case-control or case-only, and in the later case, the local ancestry of disease cases is compared with the local ancestry elsewhere in the genome.

Since the selected AIMs have high population differentiation and are unlinked in each ancestry populations, Hidden Markov model (HMM) based approaches are used to infer the local ancestry and are implemented in several software packages, including ADMIXMAP, ANCESTRYAMP and MALDsoft[181]. Using admixture mapping, many complex diseases associated loci have been identified by selected AIMs[99, 182-184]. For example, admixture mapping identifies 8q24 as a prostate cancer risk locus in African-American men, which can be replicated by later GWAS[185]. However, admixture mappings based on economic AIMs do not account for high-LD between markers, which makes it less powerful than studies inferring local ancestry based on genome-wide high-density data[181]. In recent years, various methods such as SABER[186], HAPAA[187] and HAPMIX[188] have been developed to infer locus-specific ancestry based on high density SNPs data. Especially, HAPMIX employs an explicit population genetic model to infer local ancestry based on fine-scale variation data for populations formed by two-way admixture[188]. HAPMIX permits small rates of miscopying from the ancestral haplotype, modeling unphased diploid data from the admixed population with the HMM. Our simulations showed that HAMPIX performed better compared with other methods when very recent admixed population were investigated[82].

6. Acknowledgements

This work was supported by the National Science Foundation of China (NSFC) grants 31171218 and 30971577, by the Shanghai Rising-Star Program 11QA1407600, and by the Science Foundation of the Chinese Academy of Sciences (CAS) (KSCX2-EW-Q-1-11; KSCX2-EW-R-01-05; KSCX2-EW-J-15-05). This research was supported in part by the Ministry of Science and Technology (MoST) International Cooperation Base of China. Shuhua Xu is Max-Planck Independent Research Group Leader and member of CAS Youth Innovation Promotion Association. Shuhua Xu also gratefully acknowledges the support of K.C.Wong Education Foundation, Hong Kong.

7. References

[1] Clark, A.G., et al., *Ascertainment bias in studies of human genome-wide polymorphism.* Genome Res, 2005. 15(11): p. 1496-502.

[2] Shendure, J. and H. Ji, *Next-generation DNA sequencing.* Nat Biotechnol, 2008. 26(10): p. 1135-45.
[3] Reich, D.E., et al., *Human genome sequence variation and the influence of gene history, mutation and recombination.* Nat Genet, 2002. 32(1): p. 135-42.
[4] Feuk, L., A.R. Carson, and S.W. Scherer, *Structural variation in the human genome.* Nat Rev Genet, 2006. 7(2): p. 85-97.
[5] Durbin, R.M., et al., *A map of human genome variation from population-scale sequencing.* Nature, 2010. 467(7319): p. 1061-73.
[6] Przeworski, M. and J.K. Pritchard, *Linkage disequilibrium in humans: Models and data.* Am J of Hum Genet, 2001. 69(1): p. 1-14.
[7] Lewontin, R.C., *Interaction of Selection + Linkage .2. Optimum Models.* Genetics, 1964. 50(4): p. 757-&.
[8] Lewontin, R.C., *Interaction of Selection + Linkage .I. General Considerations - Heterotic Models.* Genetics, 1964. 49(1): p. 49-&.
[9] Frazer, K.A., et al., *A second generation human haplotype map of over 3.1 million SNPs.* Nature, 2007. 449(7164): p. 851-61.
[10] Altshuler, D., et al., *A haplotype map of the human genome.* Nature, 2005. 437(7063): p. 1299-1320.
[11] Rosenberg, N.A., et al., *A worldwide survey of haplotype variation and linkage disequilibrium in the human genome.* Nat Genet, 2006. 38(11): p. 1251-1260.
[12] Xu, S. and L. Jin, *Chromosome-wide haplotype sharing: a measure integrating recombination information to reconstruct the phylogeny of human populations.* Ann Hum Genet, 2011. 75(6): p. 694-706.
[13] Kong, A., et al., *A high-resolution recombination map of the human genome.* Nat Genet, 2002. 31(3): p. 241-7.
[14] Kauppi, L., A.J. Jeffreys, and S. Keeney, *Where the crossovers are: recombination distributions in mammals.* Nat Rev Genet, 2004. 5(6): p. 413-24.
[15] Nordborg M: *Coalescent theory.* In Handbook of Statistical Genetics. Edited by Balding DJ, Bishop M, Cannings C. Chichester, UK: John Wiley & Sons Inc; 2001:p. 179-212.
[16] Wakeley, J. 2008. Coalescent Theory: *An Introduction.* Roberts & Co , Greenwood Village, Colorado.
[17] Wiuf, C. and J. Hein, *Recombination as a point process along sequences.* Theor Popul Biol, 1999. 55(3): p. 248-259.
[18] Wiuf, C. and J. Hein, *The ancestry of a sample of sequences subject to recombination.* Genetics, 1999. 151(3): p. 1217-28.
[19] Griffiths, R.C. and P. Marjoram, *Ancestral inference from samples of DNA sequences with recombination.* J Comput Biol, 1996. 3(4): p. 479-502.
[20] Stumpf, M.P. and G.A. McVean, *Estimating recombination rates from population-genetic data.* Nat Rev Genet, 2003. 4(12): p. 959-68.
[21] Coop, G., et al., *High-resolution mapping of crossovers reveals extensive variation in fine-scale recombination patterns among humans.* Science, 2008. 319(5868): p. 1395-8.
[22] McVean, G.A.T., et al., *The fine-scale structure of recombination rate variation in the human genome.* Science, 2004. 304(5670): p. 581-584.
[23] Posada, D. and K.A. Crandall, *Evaluation of methods for detecting recombination from DNA sequences: computer simulations.* Proc Natl Acad Sci U S A, 2001. 98(24): p. 13757-62.
[24] Wang, Y. and B. Rannala, *Population genomic inference of recombination rates and hotspots.* Proc Natl Acad Sci U S A, 2009. 106(15): p. 6215-6219.
[25] Rannala, B. and Y. Wang, *Bayesian inference of fine-scale recombination rates using population genomic data.* Phil Trans R Soc B, 2008. 363(1512): p. 3921-3930.

[26] Fearnhead, P. and P. Donnelly, *Approximate likelihood methods for estimating local recombination rates.* J R Stat Soc B, 2002. 64: p. 657-680.

[27] Hudson, R.R., *Two-locus sampling distributions and their application.* Genetics, 2001. 159(4): p. 1805-1817.

[28] Donnelly, P., et al., *A fine-scale map of recombination rates and hotspots across the human genome.* Science, 2005. 310(5746): p. 321-324.

[29] Wegmann, D., et al., *Recombination rates in admixed individuals identified by ancestry-based inference.* Nat Genet, 2011. 43(9): p. 847-53.

[30] Hinch, A.G., et al., *The landscape of recombination in African Americans.* Nature, 2011. 476(7359): p. 170-5.

[31] Wang, J., *Estimation of effective population sizes from data on genetic markers.* Philos Trans R Soc Lond B Biol Sci, 2005. 360(1459): p. 1395-409.

[32] Hill, W.G., *Estimation of Effective Population-Size from Data on Linkage Disequilibrium.* Genet Res, 1981. 38(3): p. 209-216.

[33] Hayes, B.J., et al., *Novel multilocus measure of linkage disequilibrium to estimate past effective population size.* Genome Res, 2003. 13(4): p. 635-643.

[34] Li, H. and R. Durbin, *Inference of human population history from individual whole-genome sequences.* Nature, 2011. 475(7357): p. 493-6.

[35] McVean, G.A. and N.J. Cardin, *Approximating the coalescent with recombination.* Philos Trans R Soc Lond B Biol Sci, 2005. 360(1459): p. 1387-93.

[36] Hey, J., *Isolation with migration models for more than two populations.* Mol Biol Evol, 2010. 27(4): p. 905-20.

[37] McHenry, H.M., *Human Evolution,* in *Evolution: The First Four Billion Years,* M.R.J. Travis, Editor. 2009, The Belknap Press of Harvard University Press: Cambridge, Massachusetts: p. 265.

[38] Cann, R.L., M. Stoneking, and A.C. Wilson, *Mitochondrial DNA and human evolution.* Nature, 1987. 325(6099): p. 31-6.

[39] Ke, Y., et al., *African origin of modern humans in East Asia: a tale of 12,000 Y chromosomes.* Science, 2001. 292(5519): p. 1151-3.

[40] Vigilant, L., et al., *African populations and the evolution of human mitochondrial DNA.* Science, 1991. 253(5027): p. 1503-7.

[41] Green, R.E., et al., *A draft sequence of the Neandertal genome.* Science, 2010. 328(5979): p. 710-22.

[42] Reich, D., et al., *Genetic history of an archaic hominin group from Denisova Cave in Siberia.* Nature, 2010. 468(7327): p. 1053-60.

[43] Reich, D., et al., *Denisova admixture and the first modern human dispersals into Southeast Asia and Oceania.* Am J Hum Genet, 2011. 89(4): p. 516-28.

[44] Rasmussen, M., et al., *An Aboriginal Australian Genome Reveals Separate Human Dispersals into Asia.* Science, 2011. 333(6052): p. 94-98.

[45] Nielsen, R., *Estimation of population parameters and recombination rates from single nucleotide polymorphisms.* Genetics, 2000. 154(2): p. 931-42.

[46] Williamson, S.H., et al., *Simultaneous inference of selection and population growth from patterns of variation in the human genome.* Proc Natl Acad Sci U S A, 2005. 102(22): p. 7882-7.

[47] Voight, B.F., et al., *Interrogating multiple aspects of variation in a full resequencing data set to infer human population size changes.* Proc Natl Acad Sci U S A, 2005. 102(51): p. 18508-13.

[48] Keinan, A., et al., *Measurement of the human allele frequency spectrum demonstrates greater genetic drift in East Asians than in Europeans.* Nat Genet, 2007. 39(10): p. 1251-5.

[49] Cavalli-Sforza, L.L., *The Human Genome Diversity Project: past, present and future.* Nat Rev Genet, 2005. 6(4): p. 333-40.
[50] Hey, J. and C.A. Machado, *The study of structured populations--new hope for a difficult and divided science.* Nat Rev Genet, 2003. 4(7): p. 535-43.
[51] Falush, D., M. Stephens, and J.K. Pritchard, *Inference of population structure using multilocus genotype data: linked loci and correlated allele frequencies.* Genetics, 2003. 164(4): p. 1567-87.
[52] Pritchard, J.K., M. Stephens, and P. Donnelly, *Inference of population structure using multilocus genotype data.* Genetics, 2000. 155(2): p. 945-59.
[53] Rosenberg, N.A., et al., *Genetic structure of human populations.* Science, 2002. 298(5602): p. 2381-5.
[54] Tang, H., et al., *Estimation of individual admixture: analytical and study design considerations.* Genet epidemiol, 2005. 28(4): p. 289-301.
[55] Pool, J.E., et al., *Population genetic inference from genomic sequence variation.* Genome Res, 2010. 20(3): p. 291-300.
[56] Li, J.Z., et al., *Worldwide human relationships inferred from genome-wide patterns of variation.* Science, 2008. 319(5866): p. 1100-4.
[57] Menozzi, P., A. Piazza, and L. Cavalli-Sforza, *Synthetic maps of human gene frequencies in Europeans.* Science, 1978. 201(4358): p. 786-92.
[58] Patterson, N., A.L. Price, and D. Reich, *Population structure and eigenanalysis.* Plos Genet, 2006. 2(12): p. e190.
[59] McVean, G., *A Genealogical Interpretation of Principal Components Analysis.* Plos Genet, 2009. 5(10).
[60] Reich, D., A.L. Price, and N. Patterson, *Principal component analysis of genetic data.* Nat Genet, 2008. 40(5): p. 491-2.
[61] Semino, O., et al., *Origin, diffusion, and differentiation of Y-chromosome haplogroups E and J: inferences on the neolithization of Europe and later migratory events in the Mediterranean area.* Am J Hum Genet, 2004. 74(5): p. 1023-34.
[62] Novembre, J. and M. Stephens, *Interpreting principal component analyses of spatial population genetic variation.* Nat Genet, 2008. 40(5): p. 646-9.
[63] Novembre, J., et al., *Genes mirror geography within Europe.* Nature, 2008. 456(7219): p. 274.
[64] Pool, J.E. and R. Nielsen, *Inference of historical changes in migration rate from the lengths of migrant tracts.* Genetics, 2009. 181(2): p. 711-9.
[65] Li, N. and M. Stephens, *Modeling linkage disequilibrium and identifying recombination hotspots using single-nucleotide polymorphism data.* Genetics, 2003. 165(4): p. 2213-33.
[66] Hellenthal, G., A. Auton, and D. Falush, *Inferring human colonization history using a copying model.* PLoS Genet, 2008. 4(5): p. e1000078.
[67] Davison, D., J.K. Pritchard, and G. Coop, *An approximate likelihood for genetic data under a model with recombination and population splitting.* Theor Popul Biol, 2009. 75(4): p. 331-45.
[68] Xu, S., W. Jin, and L. Jin, *Haplotype-sharing analysis showing Uyghurs are unlikely genetic donors.* Mol Biol Evol, 2009. 26(10): p. 2197-206.
[69] HUGO Pan-Asian SNP Consortium, et al., *Mapping human genetic diversity in Asia.* Science, 2009. 326(5959): p. 1541-5.
[70] Sabeti, P.C., et al., *Positive natural selection in the human lineage.* Science, 2006. 312(5780): p. 1614-20.
[71] Akey, J.M., *Constructing genomic maps of positive selection in humans: where do we go from here?* Genome Res, 2009. 19(5): p. 711-22.

[72] Stajich, J.E. and M.W. Hahn, *Disentangling the effects of demography and selection in human history*. Mol Biol Evol, 2005. 22(1): p. 63-73.
[73] Kimura, M., *The neutral theory of molecular evolution.* (United Kingdom: Cambridge University Press, Cambridge), 2003.
[74] Sabeti, P.C., et al., *Detecting recent positive selection in the human genome from haplotype structure.* Nature, 2002. 419(6909): p. 832-837.
[75] Tang, K., K.R. Thornton, and M. Stoneking, *A new approach for using genome scans to detect recent positive selection in the human genome*. Plos Biol, 2007. 5(7): p. 1587-1602.
[76] Voight, B.F., et al., *A map of recent positive selection in the human genome.* Plos Biol, 2006. 4(3): p. 446-458.
[77] Sabeti, P.C., et al., *Genome-wide detection and characterization of positive selection in human populations*. Nature, 2007. 449(7164): p. 913-8.
[78] Weir, B.S. and C.C. Cockerham, *Estimating F-statistics for the analysis of population structure.* Evolution, 1984. 38(6): p. 1358-1370.
[79] Akey, J.M., et al., *Interrogating a high-density SNP map for signatures of natural selection.* Genome Res, 2002. 12(12): p. 1805.
[80] Xu, S., et al., *A genome-wide search for signals of high-altitude adaptation in Tibetans.* Mol Biol Evol, 2011. 28(2): p. 1003-11.
[81] Chen, H., N. Patterson, and D. Reich, *Population differentiation as a test for selective sweeps.* Genome Res, 2010. 20(3): p. 393-402.
[82] Jin, W., et al., *Genome-wide detection of natural selection in African Americans pre- and post-admixture.* Genome Res, 2011. doi:10.1101/gr.124784.111.
[83] Long, J.C., *The genetic structure of admixed populations.* Genetics, 1991. 127(2): p. 417-28.
[84] Tang, H., et al., *Recent genetic selection in the ancestral admixture of Puerto Ricans.* Am J Hum Genet, 2007. 81(3): p. 626-33.
[85] Grossman, S.R., et al., A *Composite of Multiple Signals Distinguishes Causal Variants in Regions of Positive Selection*. Science, 2010. 327(5967): p. 883-886.
[86] Hernandez, R.D., et al., *Classic selective sweeps were rare in recent human evolution.* Science, 2011. 331(6019): p. 920-4.
[87] Tattersall, I., *Human origins: Out of Africa.* Proc Natl Acad Sci U S A, 2009. 106(38): p. 16018-16021.
[88] Pickrell, J.K., et al., *Signals of recent positive selection in a worldwide sample of human populations.* Genome Res, 2009. 19(5): p. 826-37.
[89] Novembre, J. and A. Di Rienzo, *Spatial patterns of variation due to natural selection in humans.* Nat Rev Genet, 2009. 10(11): p. 745-55.
[90] Balaresque, P.L., S.J. Ballereau, and M.A. Jobling, *Challenges in human genetic diversity: demographic history and adaptation.* Hum Mol Genet, 2007. 16 (R2): p. R134-9.
[91] Katzmarzyk, P.T. and W.R. Leonard, *Climatic influences on human body size and proportions: Ecological adaptations and secular trends.* Am J of Phys Anthropol, 1998. 106(4): p. 483-503.
[92] Parra, E.J., *Human pigmentation variation: Evolution, genetic basis, and implications for public health.* Am J of Phys Anthropol, 2007: p. 85-105.
[93] Jablonski, N.G. and G. Chaplin, *Human skin pigmentation as an adaptation to UV radiation.* Proc Natl Acad Sci U S A, 2010. 107: p. 8962-8968.
[94] Harding, R.M., et al., *Evidence for variable selective pressures at MC1R.* Am J Hum Genet, 2000. 66(4): p. 1351-61.
[95] Norton, H.L., et al., *Genetic evidence for the convergent evolution of light skin in Europeans and East Asians*. Mol Biol Evol, 2007. 24(3): p. 710-22.

[96] Calvo, M.S., S.J. Whiting, and C.N. Barton, *Vitamin D intake: a global perspective of current status.* J Nutr, 2005. 135(2): p. 310-6.
[97] Young, J.H., et al., *Differential susceptibility to hypertension is due to selection during the out-of-Africa expansion.* PLoS Genet, 2005. 1(6): p. e82.
[98] Kurian, A.K. and K.M. *Cardarelli, Racial and ethnic differences in cardiovascular disease risk factors: a systematic review.* Ethn Dis, 2007. 17(1): p. 143-52.
[99] Zhu, X., et al., *Admixture mapping for hypertension loci with genome-scan markers.* Nat Genet, 2005. 37(2): p. 177-81.
[100] Moore, L.G., *Human genetic adaptation to high altitude.* High Alt Med Biol, 2001. 2(2): p. 257-79.
[101] Bigham, A., et al., *Identifying Signatures of Natural Selection in Tibetan and Andean Populations Using Dense Genome Scan Data.* Plos Genet, 2010. 6(9).
[102] Beall, C.M., et al., *Hemoglobin concentration of high-altitude Tibetans and Bolivian Aymara.* Am J of Phys Anthropol, 1998. 106(3): p. 385-400.
[103] Zhuang, J., et al., *Hypoxic ventilatory responsiveness in Tibetan compared with Han residents of 3,658 m.* J Appl Physiol, 1993. 74(1): p. 303-11.
[104] Yi, X., et al., *Sequencing of 50 human exomes reveals adaptation to high altitude.* Science, 2010. 329(5987): p. 75-8.
[105] Simonson, T.S., et al., *Genetic evidence for high-altitude adaptation in Tibet.* Science, 2010. 329(5987): p. 72-5.
[106] Perry, G.H., et al., *Diet and the evolution of human amylase gene copy number variation.* Nat Genet, 2007. 39(10): p. 1256-60.
[107] Diamond, J., *Evolution, consequences and future of plant and animal domestication.* Nature, 2002. 418(6898): p. 700-7.
[108] Cordain, L., et al., *Origins and evolution of the Western diet: health implications for the 21st century.* Am J Clin Nutr, 2005. 81(2): p. 341-354.
[109] Neel, J.V., Diabetes mellitus: a "thrifty" genotype rendered detrimental by "progress"? Am J Hum Genet, 1962. 14: p. 353-62.
[110] Eaton, S.B., M. Konner, and M. Shostak, *Stone agers in the fast lane: chronic degenerative diseases in evolutionary perspective.* Am J Med, 1988. 84(4): p. 739-49.
[111] Helgason, A., et al., *Refining the impact of TCF7L2 gene variants on type 2 diabetes and adaptive evolution.* Nat Genet, 2007. 39(2): p. 218-25.
[112] Peltonen, L., et al., *Identification of a variant associated with adult-type hypolactasia.* Nat Genet, 2002. 30(2): p. 233-237.
[113] Swallow, D.M., *Genetics of lactase persistence and lactose intolerance.* Annu Rev Genet, 2003. 37: p. 197-219.
[114] Wang, Y.X., et al., *The Lactase Persistence/Non-Persistence Polymorphism Is Controlled by a Cis-Acting Element.* Hum Mol Genet, 1995. 4(4): p. 657-662.
[115] Bersaglieri, T., et al., *Genetic signatures of strong recent positive selection at the lactase gene.* Am J Hum Genet, 2004. 74(6): p. 1111-20.
[116] Poulter, M., et al., *The causal element for the lactase persistence/non-persistence polymorphism is located in a 1 Mb region of linkage disequilibrium in Europeans.* Ann of Hum Genet, 2003. 67: p. 298-311.
[117] Tishkoff, S.A., et al., *Convergent adaptation of human lactase persistence in Africa and Europe.* Nat Genet, 2007. 39(1): p. 31-40.
[118] Casanova, J.L. and L. Abel, *Inborn errors of immunity to infection: the rule rather than the exception.* J Exp Med, 2005. 202(2): p. 197-201.
[119] Haldane, J.B.S., *Disease and Evolution* (Reprinted from La Ricerca Scientifica Supplemento, Vol 19, Pg 1-11, 1949). Curr Sci, 1992. 63(9-10): p. 599-604.

[120] Varki, A., *A chimpanzee genome project is a biomedical imperative.* Genome Res, 2000. 10(8): p. 1065-1070.

[121] Varki, A. and T.K. Altheide, *Comparing the human and chimpanzee genomes: Searching for needles in a haystack.* Genome Res, 2005. 15(12): p. 1746-1758.

[122] Sironi, M., et al., *Widespread balancing selection and pathogen-driven selection at blood group antigen genes.* Genome Res, 2009. 19(2): p. 199-212.

[123] Prugnolle, F., et al., *Pathogen-driven selection and worldwide HLA class I diversity.* Curr Biol, 2005. 15(11): p. 1022-1027.

[124] Barreiro, L.B. and L. Quintana-Murci, *From evolutionary genetics to human immunology: how selection shapes host defence genes.* Nat Rev Genet, 2010. 11(1): p. 17-30.

[125] Moyzis, R.K., et al., *Global landscape of recent inferred Darwinian selection for Homo sapiens.* Proc Natl Acad Sci U S A, 2006. 103(1): p. 135-140.

[126] Wolfe, N.D., C.P. Dunavan, and J. Diamond, *Origins of major human infectious diseases.* Nature, 2007. 447(7142): p. 279-83.

[127] Barreiro, L.B., et al., *Evolutionary Dynamics of Human Toll-Like Receptors and Their Different Contributions to Host Defense.* Plos Genet, 2009. 5(7).

[128] Casanova, J.L., et al., *Immunology in natura: clinical, epidemiological and evolutionary genetics of infectious diseases.* Nat Immunol, 2007. 8(11): p. 1165-1171.

[129] Arenzana-Seisdedos, F. and M. Parmentier, *Genetics of resistance to HIV infection: Role of co-receptors and co-receptor ligands.* Seminars in Immunology, 2006. 18(6): p. 387-403.

[130] Galvani, A.P. and M. Slatkin, *Evaluating plague and smallpox as historical selective pressures for the CCR5-Delta 32 HIV-resistance allele.* Proc Natl Acad Sci U S A, 2003. 100(25): p. 15276-15279.

[131] Snow, R.W., et al., *The global distribution of clinical episodes of Plasmodium falciparum malaria.* Nature, 2005. 434(7030): p. 214-217.

[132] Kwiatkowski, D.P., *How malaria has affected the human genome and what human genetics can teach us about malaria.* Am J Hum Genet, 2005. 77(2): p. 171-192.

[133] Schork, N.J., et al., *Common vs. rare allele hypotheses for complex diseases.* Curr Opin Genet Dev, 2009. 19(3): p. 212-9.

[134] Luo, L., E. Boerwinkle, and M. Xiong, *Association studies for next-generation sequencing.* Genome Res, 2011. 21(7): p. 1099-108.

[135] Di Rienzo, A. and R.R. Hudson, *An evolutionary framework for common diseases: the ancestral-susceptibility model.* Trends Genet, 2005. 21(11): p. 596-601.

[136] Di Rienzo, A., *Population genetics models of common diseases.* Curr Opi Genet Dev, 2006. 16(6): p. 630-636.

[137] Pritchard, J.K., *Are rare variants responsible for susceptibility to complex diseases?* Am J Hum Genet, 2001. 69(1): p. 124-137.

[138] Kryukov, G.V., L.A. Pennacchio, and S.R. Sunyaev, *Most rare missense alleles are deleterious in humans: implications for complex disease and association studies.* Am J Hum Genet, 2007. 80(4): p. 727-39.

[139] Hindorff, L.A., et al., *Potential etiologic and functional implications of genome-wide association loci for human diseases and traits.* Proc Natl Acad Sci U S A, 2009. 106(23): p. 9362-7.

[140] McCarthy, M.I., et al., *Genome-wide association studies for complex traits: consensus, uncertainty and challenges.* Nat Rev Genet, 2008. 9(5): p. 356-369.

[141] Reich, D.E. and E.S. Lander, *On the allelic spectrum of human disease.* Trends Genet, 2001. 17(9): p. 502-10.

[142] Bodmer, W. and C. Bonilla, *Common and rare variants in multifactorial susceptibility to common diseases.* Nat Genet, 2008. 40(6): p. 695-701.

[143] Gibson, G., *Decanalization and the origin of complex disease.* Nat Rev Genet, 2009. 10(2): p. 134-40.
[144] Hermisson, J. and G.P. Wagner, *The population genetic theory of hidden variation and genetic robustness. Genetics*, 2004. 168(4): p. 2271-84.
[145] Polychronakos, C., *Common and rare alleles as causes of complex phenotypes.* Curr Atheroscler Rep, 2008. 10(3): p. 194-200.
[146] Dickson, S.P., et al., *Rare variants create synthetic genome-wide associations.* PLoS Biol, 2010. 8(1): p. e1000294.
[147] Romeo, S., et al., *Population-based resequencing of ANGPTL4 uncovers variations that reduce triglycerides and increase HDL.* Nat Genet, 2007. 39(4): p. 513-6.
[148] Ji, W., et al., *Rare independent mutations in renal salt handling genes contribute to blood pressure variation.* Nat Genet, 2008. 40(5): p. 592-9.
[149] McCarthy, M.I., et al., *Genome-wide association studies for complex traits: consensus, uncertainty and challenges.* Nat Rev Genet, 2008. 9(5): p. 356-69.
[150] *Genome-wide association study of 14,000 cases of seven common diseases and 3,000 shared controls.* Nature, 2007. 447(7145): p. 661-78.
[151] Price, A.L., et al., *Principal components analysis corrects for stratification in genome-wide association studies.* Nat Genet, 2006. 38(8): p. 904-9.
[152] Clayton, D.G., et al., *Population structure, differential bias and genomic control in a large-scale, case-control association study.* Nat Genet, 2005. 37(11): p. 1243-6.
[153] Marchini, J., et al., *The effects of human population structure on large genetic association studies.* Nat Genet, 2004. 36(5): p. 512-7.
[154] Seldin, M.F., et al., *European population substructure: clustering of northern and southern populations.* PLoS Genet, 2006. 2(9): p. e143.
[155] Tian, C., et al., *Analysis and application of European genetic substructure using 300 K SNP information. PLoS Genet*, 2008. 4(1): p. e4.
[156] Xu, S., et al., *Genomic dissection of population substructure of Han Chinese and its implication in association studies.* Am J Hum Genet, 2009. 85(6): p. 762-74.
[157] Chen, J., et al., *Genetic structure of the Han Chinese population revealed by genome-wide SNP variation.* Am J Hum Genet, 2009. 85(6): p. 775-85.
[158] Zheng, G., B. Freidlin, and J.L. Gastwirth, *Robust genomic control for association studies.* Am J Hum Genet, 2006. 78(2): p. 350-6.
[159] Jin, W., et al., *A systematic characterization of genes underlying both complex and Mendelian diseases.* Hum Mol Genet, 2011. doi:10.1093/hmg/DDR599.
[160] Visscher, P.M., *Sizing up human height variation.* Nat Genet, 2008. 40(5): p. 489-90.
[161] Manolio, T.A., et al., *Finding the missing heritability of complex diseases.* Nature, 2009. 461(7265): p. 747-53.
[162] Ng, S.B., et al., *Targeted capture and massively parallel sequencing of 12 human exomes.* Nature, 2009. 461(7261): p. 272-6.
[163] Li, Y., et al., *Low-coverage sequencing: implications for design of complex trait association studies.* Genome Res, 2011. 21(6): p. 940-51.
[164] Gorlov, I.P., et al., *Shifting paradigm of association studies: value of rare single-nucleotide polymorphisms.* Am J Hum Genet, 2008. 82(1): p. 100-12.
[165] Li, B. and S.M. Leal, *Methods for detecting associations with rare variants for common diseases: application to analysis of sequence data.* Am J Hum Genet, 2008. 83(3): p. 311-21.
[166] Li, Y., A.E. Byrnes, and M. Li, *To identify associations with rare variants, just WHaIT: Weighted haplotype and imputation-based tests.* Am J Hum Genet, 2010. 87(5): p. 728-35.

[167] Price, A.L., et al., *Pooled association tests for rare variants in exon-resequencing studies.* Am J Hum Genet, 2010. 86(6): p. 832-8.
[168] Xu, S., et al., *Analysis of genomic admixture in Uyghur and its implication in mapping strategy.* Am J Hum Genet, 2008. 82(4): p. 883-94.
[169] Xu, S. and L. Jin, *A genome-wide analysis of admixture in Uyghurs and a high-density admixture map for disease-gene discovery.* Am J Hum Genet, 2008. 83(3): p. 322-36.
[170] Narang, A., et al., *Recent admixture in an Indian population of African ancestry.* Am J Hum Genet, 2011. 89(1): p. 111-20.
[171] Shah, A.M., et al., *Indian Siddis: African descendants with Indian admixture.* Am J Hum Genet, 2011. 89(1): p. 154-61.
[172] Smith, M.W. and S.J. O'Brien, *Mapping by admixture linkage disequilibrium: advances, limitations and guidelines.* Nat Rev Genet, 2005. 6(8): p. 623--632.
[173] Bamshad, M., et al., *Deconstructing the relationship between genetics and race.* Nat Rev Genet, 2004. 5(8): p. 598-609.
[174] Chakraborty, R. and K.M. Weiss, *Admixture as a tool for finding linked genes and detecting that difference from allelic association between loci.* Proc Natl Acad Sci U S A, 1988. 85(23): p. 9119-23.
[175] Stephens, J.C., D. Briscoe, and S.J. O'Brien, *Mapping by admixture linkage disequilibrium in human populations: limits and guidelines.* Am J Hum Genet, 1994. 55(4): p. 809-24.
[176] Pfaff, C.L., et al., *Population structure in admixed populations: effect of admixture dynamics on the pattern of linkage disequilibrium.* Am J Hum Genet, 2001. 68(1): p. 198-207.
[177] Tian, C., et al., *A genomewide single-nucleotide-polymorphism panel with high ancestry information for African American admixture mapping.* Am J Hum Genet, 2006. 79(4): p. 640-9.
[178] Pfaff, C.L., R.A. Kittles, and M.D. Shriver, *Adjusting for population structure in admixed populations.* Genet Epidemiol, 2002. 22(2): p. 196-201.
[179] Seldin, M.F., et al., *Putative ancestral origins of chromosomal segments in individual african americans: implications for admixture mapping.* Genome Res, 2004. 14(6): p. 1076-84.
[180] Xu, S., et al., *Dissecting linkage disequilibrium in African-American genomes: roles of markers and individuals.* Mol Biol Evol, 2007. 24(9): p. 2049-58.
[181] Seldin, M.F., B. Pasaniuc, and A.L. Price, *New approaches to disease mapping in admixed populations.* Nat Rev Genet, 2011. 12(8): p. 523-8.
[182] Freedman, M.L., et al., *Admixture mapping identifies 8q24 as a prostate cancer risk locus in African-American men.* Proc Natl Acad Sci U S A, 2006. 103(38): p. 14068-73.
[183] Cheng, C.-Y., et al., *Admixture mapping of 15,280 African Americans identifies obesity susceptibility loci on chromosomes 5 and X.* PLoS Genet, 2009. 5(5): p. e1000490.
[184] Reich, D., et al., *A whole-genome admixture scan finds a candidate locus for multiple sclerosis susceptibility.* Nat Genet, 2005. 37(10): p. 1113-8.
[185] Gudmundsson, J., et al., *Genome-wide association study identifies a second prostate cancer susceptibility variant at 8q24.* Nat Genet, 2007. 39(5): p. 631-7.
[186] Tang, H., et al., *Reconstructing genetic ancestry blocks in admixed individuals.* Am J Hum Genet, 2006. 79(1): p. 1-12.
[187] Sundquist, A., et al., *Effect of genetic divergence in identifying ancestral origin using HAPAA.* Genome Res, 2008. 18(4): p. 676-82.
[188] Price, A.L., et al., *Sensitive detection of chromosomal segments of distinct ancestry in admixed populations.* PLoS Genet, 2009. 5(6): p. e1000519.